Meet the editor

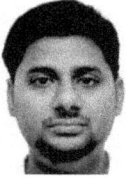

Dr. Alok Raghav obtained his Ph.D. in Endocrinology from Rajiv Gandhi Centre for Diabetes and Endocrinology, J. N. Medical College, Faculty of Medicine, Aligarh Muslim University, India. He worked as a project scientist at the Indian Institute of Technology in Kanpur, India. He has more than ten years of research experience in the field of glycobiology and diabetes mellitus. He also worked as Scientist C at the Multidisciplinary Research Unit (sponsored by the Department of Health Research, Ministry of Health and Family Welfare, New Delhi), GSVM Medical College, Kanpur, India. He is currently working as a Research Professor at the School of Medicine, Department of Anatomy & Cell Biology, Lee Gil Ya Cancer and Diabetes Institute, Gachon University, South Korea. Dr. Raghav has received several international and national awards. He is also an associate editor for Frontiers in Endocrinology and Frontiers in Public Health and an academic editor for PLOS One.

Contents

Preface

Diabetes mellitus is one of the most challenging diseases of the current century, with its link to micro-and macro-vascular complications imposing a substantial economic and health burden on the healthcare system and society. Of the associated complications, diabetic foot contributes significantly to quality-of-life impairment, hospitalization recurrences, and, in extreme cases, limb amputation. Despite recent technological developments in the medical sciences, the prevention and successful management of diabetic foot complications remain clinical, surgical, and rehabilitative challenges worldwide.

The current edited book brings together a comprehensive and detailed set of chapters contributed by specialists from various fields. The book offers a comprehensive synthesis of evidence-based interventions and emerging technologies for preventing, diagnosing, and treating diabetic foot complications. The current book is intended for a broad readership, including clinicians, scientists, allied healthcare professionals, and policymakers, to provide in-depth insights.

Particular attention is given to multidisciplinary models of care, described in chapters, highlighting the value of collaborative strategies that integrate endocrinologists, surgeons, podiatrists, nurses, and rehabilitation experts. Additionally, chapters on patient education, psychosocial factors, and community-level prevention strategies remind us that outcomes depend as much on holistic care and empowerment as on technical skills.

An especially valuable contribution to this book is the presentation of cutting-edge technologies, including regenerative medicine, bioengineered dermal substitutes, negative pressure wound therapy, and computerized tools for early detection. These topics are discussed in Chapters that, together, present the future of diabetic foot care.

In presenting such contributions, our intention is not only to provide a state-of-the-art guide to clinical practice but also to encourage enhanced research and collaboration in this important subject. The organization of the chapters has been designed to guide the reader from pathophysiologic insights to diagnostic and therapeutic modalities, and ultimately to innovative horizons, providing both coherence and substance.

We are highly appreciative of all contributing authors' dedication and expertise, without which this volume would have been impossible. Their efforts demonstrate academic rigor and a passion to improve the lives of individuals affected by diabetic foot complications. We also offer our heartfelt thanks to peer reviewers, editorial assistants, and the IntechOpen publishing team for their outstanding support in preparing this book.

Lastly, we hope this book will serve as a helpful tool for readers across fields, stimulating ongoing conversation, creativity, and enhanced patient care for individuals at risk of or with diabetic foot disease.

Alok Raghav
Gachon University,
Incheon, Republic of Korea

Section 1

Methods and Approach

Chapter 1

Introductory Chapter: Diabetic Foot – Emerging Strategies in Clinical Management

Alok Raghav

1. Introduction

Diabetic foot is a threat to society as it severely affects the patient's quality of life and poses an economic burden to healthcare. Diabetic foot includes numerous chronic complications, infections, foot ulcerations, and limb amputations. These complications significantly contribute to the mortality and morbidity of patients with diabetes. Consequently, chronic complications or diabetic foot disease are a growing concern worldwide and represent major global medical, social, and economic problems. Diabetic foot ulcers (DFU) are a major endpoint of diabetic foot disease. Peripheral nerve damage and peripheral vascular diseases are common etiological factors for DFU, which seldom present with the decreased peripheral blood flow and decreased local angiogenesis. Biochemical perturbations and a significant increase in susceptibility to infection are among the risk factors for DFU [1, 2].

2. Etiology and pathogenesis of diabetic foot

Foot ulcers in individuals with diabetes result from a multifactorial pathophysiology, primarily involving neuropathy, ischemia, and infection, which often act in synergy [3]. Peripheral neuropathy, present in nearly half of patients with diabetes, is a major contributor, as sensory loss predisposes patients to unnoticed trauma and high-pressure zones that progress to ulceration. Motor neuropathy leads to muscle atrophy, deformities, and abnormal gait, increasing plantar pressure, whereas autonomic neuropathy causes anhidrosis, skin fissures, and impaired microcirculation, further increasing the risk. Ischemia, largely due to peripheral arterial disease (PAD), plays a growing role, with studies showing that nearly half of diabetic foot ulcers (DFUs) in high-income countries are ischemic or neuro-ischemic [3]. PAD in diabetes is characterized by the multisegmented, bilateral infrapopliteal involvement with poor collateralization, which impairs healing and elevates the risk of amputation. Infection, often secondary to neuropathy and ischemia, rapidly spreads through fascial and tendon compartments and accounts for 25–50% of amputations in patients with DFUs. Additional risk factors include long-standing diabetes, male sex, poor glycemic control, renal disease, prior ulcers or amputations, and foot deformity [3]. Thus, DFU development reflects the complex interplay of neuropathy, vascular compromise, and infection, with ischemia and infection being the principal determinants of poor healing and limb loss.

IntechOpen

Approximately half of individuals with diabetes develop peripheral neuropathy within 25 years, most often distal polyneuropathy, although motor and autonomic fibers may also be involved [4]. Its severity correlates with long-term hyperglycemia, dyslipidemia, oxidative stress, and pathways such as advanced glycation, protein kinase C, and polyol pathways [4]. Peripheral vascular disease further contributes to foot ulceration through endothelial dysfunction, basement membrane thickening, impaired vasodilation, and hypercoagulability, all of which promote ischemia. In addition, hyperglycemia impairs immune function by reducing fibroblast activity, keratinocyte migration, and inflammatory response, making patients more prone to recurrent soft tissue and bone infections that worsen glycemic control [4]. Together, neuropathy, vasculopathy, and immunopathy create a vicious cycle of impaired healing, infection, and tissue breakdown, predisposing patients with diabetes to limb-threatening foot complications.

3. Clinical presentation

The diabetic foot may appear normal at first glance; however, it has distinct clinical features that can easily be overlooked. Motor neuropathy leads to atrophy of the lumbrical and interosseous muscles, resulting in clawed toes, hammertoe deformities, and prominent metatarsal heads, which create focal pressure points prone to ulceration [5]. Charcot neuroarthropathy (CN), a severe complication often associated with diabetic foot ulcers (DFU), causes progressive bone and joint destruction, and may mimic cellulitis, osteomyelitis, arthritis, or sprain, frequently leading to misdiagnosis. Early CN presents with a warm, swollen, red joint, often painless, with radiologic evidence of microfractures; advanced stages can result in midfoot collapse and rocker-bottom deformity [5]. A diabetic foot also shows dry, cracked skin, calluses, and pre-ulcerative signs such as redness, blisters, or fissures. In patients with peripheral arterial disease (PAD), the foot may appear pale and cold, although ischemia may sometimes present as warm and pink due to arteriovenous shunts or CN. Classical ischemic symptoms, such as rest pain or gangrene, may be absent. Similarly, infection signs are often masked by PAD, neuropathy, and immunopathy; redness, swelling, or fever may be minimal, and unexplained hyperglycemia may be the only indicator. Accurate ulcer assessment requires debridement to uncover hidden abscesses and deep tissue involvement [5].

4. Classification of diabetic foot

The classification of diabetic foot ulcers (DFU) is essential for guiding treatment, predicting outcomes, and enabling standardized communication; however, no universally accepted system exists. Several schemes have been developed, each with unique strengths and limitations. The Meggitt-Wagner system classifies ulcers into six grades based mainly on depth and necrosis, making it simple but limited because it does not account for ischemia or infection [6]. The University of Texas (UT) system improves this by combining ulcer depth with the presence of infection or ischemia, offering a better prognostic value for amputation. The S(AD) SAD system scores ulcers by size, infection, ischemia, and neuropathy, allowing detailed audit and research use; however, its complexity limits routine clinical application. The simplified SINBAD system grades six key elements site, ischemia, neuropathy, bacterial infection, area, and depth into a 0–6 score, balancing ease of use with robustness, and is recommended by the IWGDF for clinical and research purposes. Finally, the

WIfI system (Wound, Ischemia, foot infection) provides a structured approach to risk stratification, particularly for neuroischemic ulcers, by grading wound severity, ischemia, and infection to guide revascularization and predict amputation risk. Together, these systems highlight the multifactorial nature of DFU and the need for tailored assessment tools across different care settings [6].

5. Management

The management of diabetic foot requires a multidisciplinary approach targeting glycemic control, offloading, vascular assessment, infection control, and wound care. Adequate glycemic control (HbA1c < 6.5–7%) reduces ulcer risk, enhances healing, and lowers the amputation rate. Offloading is central to neuropathic ulcers, using devices such as total contact casts, walkers, orthoses, or surgical correction, when necessary, with patient compliance being crucial. In ischemic DFU, vascular status should be assessed (ABI, toe pressure, $TcPO_2$) and revascularization *via* endovascular therapy, bypass surgery, or emerging methods such as deep vein arterialization should be considered, especially in severe ischemia. Infection management requires antibiotics guided by tissue culture and severity; however, deep infections, necrosis, abscesses, or gangrene often necessitate surgical drainage, debridement, or even amputation, with efforts to preserve the knee joint for mobility. Local wound care, including sharp debridement and advanced dressings (hydrogels, foams, and alginates), supports healing by maintaining moisture, controlling exudate, and preventing infection, although no single dressing is superior. If standard therapy fails within 4 weeks, adjunctive options such as hyperbaric oxygen or negative pressure therapy may be used after reassessment. Overall, individualized, timely, and coordinated care is essential to improve healing, prevent recurrence, and reduce limb loss in patients with diabetes.

6. Conclusion

Diabetic foot ulcer prevention and management require a multidisciplinary approach based on the principles of education, debridement, and offloading. Preventive strategies, especially patient education and self-care, remain the cornerstones of reducing ulcer risk. Optimal glycemic control, supported by exercise, slows the progression of complications and improves healing outcomes. Offloading through total contact casts, removable walkers, or therapeutic footwear is essential, whereas surgery addresses structural deformities when conservative measures fail. Infection control with judicious antibiotic use is critical to prevent poor outcomes, and postoperative and long-term care are vital to reduce recurrence and amputation risk. Importantly, patient quality of life must be integrated into treatment planning because acceptance and adherence strongly influence outcomes. Collectively, comprehensive and individualized management combining medical, surgical, and psychosocial care offers the best chance of preventing complications, reducing amputations, and improving survival in patients with diabetic foot ulcers.

Conflict of interest

The authors declare no conflicts of interest.

Author details

Alok Raghav[1,2,3]

1 Department of Cell Biology and Anatomy, Lee Gill Ya Cancer and Diabetes Institute, Gachon University, Incheon, Republic of Korea

2 Adjunct Faculty, University Centre for Research and Development (UCRD), Chandigarh University, India

3 Adjunct Faculty, Center for Global Health Research, Saveetha Medical College and Hospital, India

*Address all correspondence to: alokalig@gmail.com; alokalig@gachon.ac.kr

IntechOpen

References

[1] Boulton AJM, Connor H, Cavanagh PR. The Pathway to Ulceration: Aetiopathogenesis. The Foot in Diabetes. 3rd ed. Chichester: John Wiley & Sons Ltd.; 2000. pp. 19-31

[2] Sinwar PD. The diabetic foot management – Recent advance. International Journal of Surgery. 2015;**15**:27-30

[3] Parveen K, Hussain MA, Anwar S, Elagib HM, Kausar MA. Comprehensive review on diabetic foot ulcers and neuropathy: Treatment, prevention and management. World Journal of Diabetes. 2025;**16**(3):100329. DOI: 10.4239/wjd.v16.i3.100329

[4] Zhu J, Hu Z, Luo Y, Liu Y, Luo W, Du X, et al. Diabetic peripheral neuropathy: Pathogenetic mechanisms and treatment. Frontiers Endocrinology. 2024;**14**:1265372. DOI: 10.3389/fendo.2023.1265372

[5] Hanna T, Latey P, Ekanayake K, Ribarovski L, McDonald R, Clarke J. Associations between diabetic foot deformity and the intrinsic foot muscles: A systematic review. Journal of Foot and Ankle Research. 2025;**18**(3):e70068. DOI: 10.1002/jfa2.70068

[6] Wang X, Yuan CX, Xu B, Yu Z. Diabetic foot ulcers: Classification, risk factors and management. World Journal of Diabetes. 2022;**13**(12):1049-1065. DOI: 10.4239/wjd.v13.i12.1049

Chapter 2

Diabetic Foot: Advanced Diagnostic and Treatment Methods

Koreyba Konstantin Aleksandrovich

Abstract

In this chapter, the author describes the pathogenetic justifications of the diagnostic algorithm in patients with diabetic foot syndrome according to the principle of "from simple to complex." Research data are available in any medical institution. Also, based on the pathogenesis of the pathological process and diagnostics, the author proposed and substantiated schemes of drug support and correction of diabetic foot syndrome at the inpatient and outpatient stages of patient care.

Keywords: pathological process of diabetic foot syndrome, diagnostic algorithm, drug correction, problematic issues of diabetic foot syndrome, local treatment

1. Introduction

DM is always associated with insulin deficiency (absolute or relative) [1]. When insulin synthesis by the B-cells of the pancreatic islet apparatus is impaired, absolute insulin deficiency develops, and when insulin metabolism is impaired, relative insulin deficiency develops. Insulin deficiency or insulin resistance in the body causes intracellular hypoglycemia and extracellular hyperglycemia. Intracellular hypoglycemia leads to fat destruction, causing diabetic ketoacidosis, and reduces the synthesis of protein and gamma globulins, causing cachexia, polyphagia, and impaired wound healing [2]. The cellular energy deficiency causes a vicarious increase in fatty acid oxidation, and the level of blood ketone bodies increases.

Imbalance of carbohydrate metabolism in diabetes mellitus: (1) decreased activity of glycolysis and adenosine triphosphate synthesis, which leads to the following events: energy deficiency, tissue hypoxia, endothelial dysfunction; (2) increased glycogenolysis, alternative glucose metabolism pathways, which lead to: hyperglycemia, polyuria, glucosuria, dehydration, and acid-electrolyte imbalance. These two points are ultimately clinically expressed in angiopathy. Protein metabolism disorder: decreased activity of the glucose metabolism pentose cycle, impaired synthesis and glycosylation of proteins, autoantibodies formation, and increased protein catabolism. This is expressed in angiopathy and neuropathy. Disruption of fat metabolism: decreased fat synthesis, activation of lipolysis, excess free fatty acids, formation of neutral fats, formation of ketones, increased formation of cholesterol, development of fatty liver infiltration, ketonemia and ketouria, development of atherosclerosis. This leads to angiopathy and endotoxicosis manifestations [3].

Thus, these three types of metabolism disorders complete the vicious circle of pathological processes. The occurrence and progression of angiopathies largely depend on oxidative stress, which occurs due to the energy impossibility of completing already started chemical reactions in cells, which leads to the death of some endothelial cells and subsequently to endothelial dysfunction.

There are only three successive natural ways for energy obtaining under aerobic conditions: glycolysis, the tricarboxylic acid cycle (Krebs cycle), and oxidative phosphorylation in the mitochondrial respiratory chain. All three are continuously employed in the body, causing the formation of carbon dioxide, water, and adenosine triphosphoric acid.

Absolute or relative insulin deficiency leads to disruption of substrate metabolism and adenosine triphosphoric acid synthesis, causing cellular starvation and energy deficiency. Under conditions of oxygen and/or blood flow deficiency (hypoxia and ischemia), the proportion of anaerobic glucose oxidation increases significantly, which is accompanied by excessive accumulation of lactate, which in turn blocks the anaerobic glycolysis reactions.

An oxidative stress is appears to be the consequence of energy deficiency, reflecting its degree and severity, that is, destructive processes occurring with the participation of an excess amount of free radicals [3].

It is oxidative stress in diabetes mellitus that leads to increased leukocyte adhesion, platelet aggregation, and disruption of endoneural blood flow, which in turn gives rise to formidable complications of this disease, that is, micro- and macroangiopathy with the subsequent retinopathy, nephropathy, encephalopathy, and neuropathy.

1.1 Endothelial dysfunction in diabetes mellitus

The main function of the circulatory system, which consists of the exchange of substances between blood and tissues, is performed by capillaries, which play the role of a histohematic barrier. The structural features of the endothelium allow dividing the capillaries into three types:

- the capillaries have a continuous endothelial lining, with no gaps in or between the cells due to indurated intercellular contacts, while the diameter of those capillaries does not exceed 10 μm, which is significantly smaller than the size of an erythrocyte; the substrates are coming from there by pinocytosis; this type of capillary forms the blood-brain barrier;

- the capillaries with tiny openings in endothelial cells, that is, pores and fenestrae (kidneys, small intestine, endocrine glands);

- the capillaries with discontinuous endothelium and basement membrane, that is, with wide intercellular gaps (liver, spleen), through which the blood counts can penetrate [3].

Angiopathies occur in almost all parts of the vasculature in diabetes mellitus. In this case, the endothelial components of the vessels are damaged first, causing a disruption of the endothelial synthesis of biologically active substances. The endocrine activity of the endothelium depends on its functional state, which is determined by the level of receipt and perception of various types of biological information. The endothelium contains numerous receptors of various biologically active substances;

it takes up pressure and volume of moving blood—the so-called fluid shear stress, stimulating the synthesis of anticoagulants and vasodilators. Biologically active substances produced by the endothelium provide both paracrine (on neighboring cells) and autocrine (on the endothelium as a whole) effects. It is worth noting that metabolic processes predominate in the endothelium of the microcirculatory bed, and metabolic and synthetic processes in the endothelium of the main vessels.

The main functions of the endothelium are the following: barrier, secretory, hemostatic, vasotonic, participation in the processes of inflammation and remodeling of the vascular wall, as well as antiatherogenic and antithrombotic. Under normal conditions, the endothelium creates an athrombogenic semipermeable barrier between blood and tissues. The barrier role of the vascular endothelium determines its main role, that is, maintaining homeostasis by regulating the equilibrium state of coagulation and fibrinolysis processes.

Disorders of any endothelial function can lead to the development of diseases, where atherosclerosis and thrombosis are the most common. In diabetes mellitus, almost all of the above-mentioned endothelial functions are deeply affected on the background of complex metabolic disorders of all types of metabolism and increasing oxidative stress, primarily the biologically active substances secreting, which is called "endothelial dysfunction" and is characterized by an imbalance between the production of vasodilating, angioprotective, antiproliferative factors on one hand and vasoconstrictive, prothrombotic and proliferative factors on the other one [3].

Recently, data on the correlation between vascular diseases and bone pathology. The individuals with low bone mineral density have hyperlipidemia and a more severe course of arterial atherosclerosis. It was established that bone and vascular tissues had a number of common morphological and molecular properties, and vascular calcification consisted of the same components as bone tissue [4]. A certain similarity in the mechanisms of osteoarthropathy and atherosclerosis development is assumed [5–7]. In the late 1990s of the twentieth century, it became known that cholesterol synthesis and osteoclast activation occur with the participation of a single cascade of biochemical processes [8]. Bone tissue and bone marrow contain endothelial cells, preosteoblasts, and osteoclasts, that is, derivatives of monocytes, and all of them are also normal components of the cellular populations of the vascular wall. In athero-sclerotic process, both bone tissue and the arterial vessel wall contain osteopontin, osteonectin, osteocalcin, bone morphogenetic protein, matrix Gla protein, collagen I, nitric oxide, and matrix vesicles. Monocytes are involved in the pathogenesis of atherosclerosis and osteoporosis, with differentiation into macrophages within the vascular wall and into osteoclasts in bone tissue. Each osteon (morphological bone unit) contains a central vessel lined with endothelium from inside which is localized on the subendothelial matrix [4].

Thus, the angiogenic damage mechanism is common in diabetes mellitus, not only causing the uniformity of clinical manifestations in pathological processes in different organs, but also dictating a unified methodology of approaches to their diagnosis and adequate therapy.

Morphologically, diabetic angiopathy is atherosclerosis with a number of features in patients with diabetes:

- more distal damage (most often the popliteal artery and leg arteries),

- bilateral and multiple localization of stenosis,

- process development at a younger age,

- comparable incidence of disease in men and women.

Osteoarthropathy does not occur in ischemia, mainly osteoporosis takes place [5].
There is a multisegmental, generalized damage of the peripheral sections of the arterial bed in diabetic atherosclerosis. The process also involves vessels located near the occlusion.

This leads to unreliability of ischemia compensation by the collateral vasculature [5]. Ischemia in diabetes progresses much faster, but pain syndrome during walking does not always occur. The pain is not characteristic of intermittent claudication syndrome. It is localized not in the lower legs, but in the feet. The equivalent of pain in diabetic foot syndrome is a feeling of weakness and fatigue of the lower leg muscles [5]. The atypism of the clinical picture is explained by the presence of diabetic polyneuropathy.

2. At the moment, the following problems still remain in the care of patients with diabetic foot syndrome

1. selection of optimal methods of medical imaging and diagnostics, with determination of further treatment tactics

2. creation of a "road map" (technology for obtaining information about the patient and treatment tactics choice), based on the diagnostic data

3. methods of general and local therapy, covering all links in the pathogenesis of diabetic foot syndrome, their stages, and timeliness

3. Diagnostic algorithm for diabetic foot syndrome

The diagnostic algorithm for the initial visit of a patient with diabetic foot syndrome begins with collecting anamnesis, complaints, and determining blood glucose levels. Then it is necessary to perform differential diagnostics of ischemic (neuroschemic) and neuropathic forms. These forms can often be distinguished by the patient's complaints.

In the neuropathic form of diabetic foot syndrome, the patients complain of dull aching pain in the feet and lower legs; the pain increases at rest and decreases with movement. Along with pain, the patients experience numbness, a crawling sensation, burning, cold, or heat in the lower extremities (paresthesia), a decrease in the pain threshold, and temperature sensitivity. Patients are often bothered by swelling of the lower legs and feet, rapid fatigue, and weakness of the leg muscles. In the neuropathic form, the foot is characterized by a deformation, the foot skin is dry, and areas of hyperkeratosis or trophic ulcers are observed in the places of excess pressure.

In the ischemic form of diabetic foot syndrome, the patients complain of intense, sharp pain in the feet and lower legs when walking (intermittent claudication), and the pain decreases at rest (when stopping). Pain at rest also occurs, especially when the patient is in a horizontal position; it decreases in a sitting and standing position. The patients often complain of rapid freezing of the feet even in summer. In the ischemic form, the skin of the foot is pale or cyanotic, atrophy and hair loss are observed, as well as ulcers on the toes and heels (acral necrosis).

3.1 Instrumental methods for diabetic neuropathy studying

Electroneuromyography is the main method for diagnosing the pathologies of nerves, muscles, peripheral motor neurons, and neuromuscular transmission. It allows identifying lesions of the neuromuscular apparatus (neural, primary muscular, and anterior horn). For polyneuropathy diagnosis, the most informative is stimulation electroneuromyography with a study of the speed of impulse conduction along motor and/or sensory fibers, and an assessment of the parameters of the obtained M-response.

3.2 Diagnosis of neuroischemic form of diabetic foot syndrome

Determination of the nature of the arterial vessel damage and the severity of ischemia is the primary diagnostic task; it is necessary to decide on the possibility and expediency of vascular reconstructive surgery.

The ankle-brachial index is important in diagnostics and prognostication of diabetic foot syndrome. It should be noted that in some patients, it may be falsely increased due to calcification of the arterial wall (Mönckeberg's medial calcific sclerosis).

Real-time ultrasound investigation (B-mode) allows visualization of stationary structures: vessel lumen and walls, surrounding tissues, and pathological processes.

Based on the reflection of ultrasonic waves from moving objects, ultrasound Doppler sonography allows obtaining quantitative, qualitative, and graphic data about blood flow physiology.

Duplex scanning allows visualization of ultrasound waves reflected from stationary objects, with the minimum diameter of the examined artery of 1 mm.

Color Doppler flow mapping by velocity allows obtaining an image in gray tones (stationary objects with resulting color mapping), which indicates the frequency shift (blood flow). A positive shift is shown in red and a negative one in blue. Turbulence looks like a mixture of red and blue spots. Color Doppler mapping allows obtaining data on the intensity and energy of blood flow, including in small vessels, where the blood velocity is lower. One of the most important characteristics of the state of the foot vascular bed in DFS (diabetic foot syndrome) is the oxygen saturation of arterial blood. It can be determined by pulse oximetry, performed using a pulse oximeter, which is based on the ability of hemoglobin, bound and not bound with oxygen, to absorb light of different wavelengths. A hemoglobin molecule can bind four O_2 molecules; the average percentage of red blood cell saturation with oxygen is called saturation. The saturation index (blood oxygen saturation level) is the ratio of the amount of hemoglobin bound with oxygen to total hemoglobin content, expressed as a percentage.

If hemoglobin bound all four O_2 molecules, then SpO_2 = 100%.

In the normal condition, the SpO_2 level shall be above 95%.

Pulse oximetry data allow the indirect determination of the partial O_2 blood pressure (paO_2), which normally equals 80–100 mm Hg. A drop in paO_2 is accompanied by a drop in blood oxygen saturation level:

- 80–100 mm Hg of paO_2 corresponds to 95–100% of the blood oxygen saturation level;

- 60 mm Hg of paO_2 corresponds to 90% of the blood oxygen saturation level;

- 40 mmHg of paO_2 corresponds to 75% of the blood oxygen saturation level.

However, it should be noted that the saturation level may be normal even in the absence of pulsation above the main arteries in hemodynamically significant stenosis, which is associated with the collateral bed activity.

For this very reason it is better to use transcutaneous oximetry to obtain accurate information about the oxygen content in the foot tissues.

The $TcpO_2$ parameter has a high prognostic value as of the outcome of neuroischemic chronic ulcers, assessment of the amputation level and wound healing. If $TcpO_2$ on the foot is more than 40 mm Hg, then the prognosis is favorable, if less than 30 mm Hg—unfavorable. A drop in the dynamics of the $TcpO_2$ parameter below 30 mm Hg is a manifestation of the increasing the degree of the main blood flow disturbance and increases the probability of amputation.

Skin tissue perfusion, detectable by laser Doppler flowmetry in patients with DFS, shows the same trends. Decreased perfusion with unchanged main blood flow in the foot, occasionally encountered in the neuroischemic form, can be explained by massive microthrombosis in the microcirculatory bed, usually accompanied by the occurrence of wet necrosis of soft tissues.

Conclusion on the possibility of vascular reconstruction of arteries and the most accurate information on the state of the vessels is provided by angiography with contrast of the distal arterial bed. X-ray contrast angiography of the lower extremities remains the "gold standard" for the diagnosis of peripheral arteries pathology. The method allows detecting the signs and the degree of stenosis and occlusion of arteries, unevenness of their contours and the level of vessel narrowing.

Diabetic macroangiopathy manifests itself in polysegmental stenoses of the arteries of the leg and foot with extended occlusions, atherosclerotic thickening of the arteries middle layer with rigidity of the vascular wall (fragility of arteries). Distal stenoses complicate carrying both endovascular and open angiosurgical operations. Extended stenoses make balloon angioplasty nearly impossible. In these patients the postoperative period is often complicated by thrombosis of bypasses, angioplasty and wound abscesses. This is usually associated with severe damage to the endothelial lining of the arteries, direct stimulating contact of platelets with the collagen of the vascular wall, and incomplete diagnostics of the grade of diabetic angio- and polyneuropathy in the preoperative period.

Despite the diagnostic value of X-ray contrast angiography, the method can cause a number of complications in patients with diabetes mellitus (severe reactions to contrast agents, contrast-induced nephropathy, which can lead to acute renal failure). That is why, to prevent these complications, all patients with diabetic foot syndrome receive perioperative hydration with isotonic solutions of sodium chloride or sodium bicarbonate with round-the-clock monitoring of diuresis, glycemia and glucosuria.

Multispiral computer-tomographic angiography is simple and fast to carry out. The contrast is iodine-containing solutions, which also provide a nephrotoxic effect.

Magnetic resonance angiography is currently a competing method with X-ray contrast angiography, since it also allows visualization of the vessels state (three-dimensional, which can be rotated), but may not require contrast (time-of-flight technique, T1 mode) or use additional contrast of the vessels. Contrast magnetic resonance angiography allows visualization of more vessels of the foot (in comparison with X-ray contrast angiography). It is worth noting, that one of the disadvantages of magnetic resonance angiography is that it cannot be performed on patients with stents, pacemakers, certain types of prostheses, etc.

3.3 Radiographic methods for assessing changes in bones and joints

In clinical practice, radiographic methods for assessing patients with DFS remain the most common, and in the case of an infected foot, they are mandatory for detecting bone damage and the development of osteomyelitis (involvement of the bone and bone marrow in the process). Bone and joint changes in diabetes mellitus are most often localized in the tarsus area. They are represented by destruction, osteolysis, bone fragmentation, osteosclerosis, and destruction of articular cartilage with narrowing of the joint space up to ankylosis. Initial manifestations of osteoarthropathy can occur with preserved blood flow and without pain, wherein swelling (edema) of the foot and individual joints, gait disturbance, and less often crepitus during movement are detected. Deformation of the longitudinal arch of the foot leads to a typical picture of a rocker bottom foot, and it is in this case that large trophic ulcers often form.

The final method for osteomyelitis diagnosing is histological examination, the material for which is most often obtained in surgery.

Thus, the decision on the form of diabetic foot syndrome is based on a neurological examination and the results of instrumental research methods (see above) of sensitivity and the condition of the main feet arteries.

Based on the above, the following practically significant and accessible examination program is proposed (from simple to complex principle):

1. In all patients at each consultation

   - palpatory study of the pulsation in the main arteries of the lower extremities

   - assessment of neurological deficit using the NDS scale (Neuropathic Dysfunction Score)

   - glycemic profile and determination of glycosylated hemoglobin level

   - pulse oximetry (oxygen saturation/SpO_2 measurement)

   - blood creatinine level, glomerular filtration rate calculation

2. In patients with revealed signs of angiopathy

   - ultrasound Doppler sonography of the arteries of the lower extremities

   - transcutaneous oximetry ($TcpO_2$)

   - consultation with a vascular surgeon to select the patient management tactics and determine indications for vascular correction

   - all patients admitted for vascular reconstruction of arteries undergo an angiographic examination (contrast or carboxyangiography)

3. In patients with foot deformities and severe hyperkeratosis

- X-ray of feet

- electroneuromyography

4. In patients with ulcerative defects of feet

- microbiological examination of wound discharge (culture)

- X-ray of feet (in case of foot deformity and/or ulcerative defects of grade 2 and grater by the Wagner classification)

After carrying out the diagnostic stage described above, all patients are recommended to be divided into four groups

1. SpO_2 monitoring values are equal to or lower than 90% and no pulsation was detected by palpation in the main arteries of the lower extremities. The patient is referred for consultation to a vascular surgeon without additional examination methods to select further diagnostic and treatment tactics.

2. SpO_2 monitoring values are equal to or below 90%, but pulsation in the main arteries of the lower limb was palpated. The patient is referred for color duplex scanning of the lower limb arteries. After that, a consultation with a vascular surgeon is possible, if necessary (this pattern may correspond to Mönckeberg's sclerosis, the etiological factor of which is diabetic neuropathy).

3. SpO_2 monitoring values are equal to or higher than 90%, and pulsation in the main arteries of the lower limb was palpated. This is evidence of the neurotrophic form of DFS. The patient is referred for feet radiography, if there are skin and soft tissue defects and/or feet deformations. Doppler ultrasound was performed in some patients to identify a correlation with pulse oximetry.

4. SpO_2 monitoring values are equal to or higher than 90%, pulsation in main arteries of the lower limb was not palpated. This diagnostic pattern is typical for atherosclerotic arterial lesions and high SpO_2 values are provided by developed collateral circulation. The patient is referred for consultation with a vascular surgeon, with parallel ultrasound Doppler sonography.

After consultation of a vascular surgeon/endovascular surgeon the patients were in turn divided into two streams after angiography:

1. Patients admitted for arterial reconstruction of arteries of the lower extremities.

2. Patients for whom reconstructive surgery on main arteries of the extremities is technically impossible due to occlusion of the distal arterial bed and patients with severe concomitant pathology (cardiovascular pathology: acute myocardial infarction, widespread post-infarction cardiosclerosis, chronic heart failure with low cardiac ejection fraction).

4. DFS pathogenetic treatment principles

- Restoration of vascular patency. Improvement of microcirculation conditions

- Prevention and relief of polyneuropathies

- Improvement of metabolic conditions and increase of tissue resistance to ischemia

- Antibacterial therapy, if an infection occurs

- Local treatment

    a. detersion of the ulcer defect from devitalized tissue

    b. closure of ulcer defect

    c. creation of favorable conditions for wound process

Taking into account the pathogenesis of pathological changes in DFS and focusing on the recommendations of expert groups at the European Association for the Study of Diabetes and national standards and clinical guidelines for providing medical care to the patients with DFS, we proposed and apply in practice several basic designs of "maintenance" drug therapy in this group of patients together with hypoglycemic therapy (patent for invention No. 2549459 of 30.03.2015 of ROSPATENT FGU FIPS RF).

4.1 Design No. 1

It is used for chronic lower limb ischemia of I–II A–B stage (according to the Fontaine-A.V. Pokrovsky scale of chronic arterial insufficiency) and clinical manifestation of diabetic polyneuropathy; if there are no indications for reconstructive surgery on the arteries of the lower limbs.

1. Antioxidants, succinic acid i.v. (slow infusion) or thioctic acid + B vitamins

2. Nicergoline

3. Pentoxifylline (*extremely careful! retinopathy! myocardial steal syndrome*)

4. Gabapentins for pain/seizure syndrome before bed

5. NSAIDs

6. Antiplatelet agents (cilostazol)

7. Antibacterial drugs, taking into account the microflora sensitivity

4.2 Design No. 2

It is used in:

1. chronic ischemia of the lower extremities of II–IV stage (according to the Fontaine-Leriche-Pokrovsky scale of chronic arterial insufficiency),

2. perioperative period, in patients administrated reconstructive vascular surgery on the lower extremities (a more pronounced clinical effect was obtained when using this design in the preoperative period),

3. critical ischemia when it is impossible to perform surgical vascular correction on the arteries of the lower extremities.

- Prostaglandins E1 in 0,9% NaCl solution, slow drip infusion during 3–4 hours

- Antioxidants, succinic acid preparations intravenously (slow infusion), nicergoline

- Thrombolytics

- Gabapentins for pain/seizure syndrome

- NSAIDs for pain syndrome

- Anticoagulants (low molecular weight heparins/rivaroxaban)

- Antiplatelet agents (cilostazol or clopidogrel + acetylsalicylic acid)

- Antibacterial drugs, considering the microflora sensitivity

Drug therapy as day hospital/outpatient and in perioperative period in arterial reconstruction

1. Antioxidants, succinic acid, thioctic acid, nicergoline

2. Clopidogrel + acetylsalicylic acid in the perioperative period for arterial reconstruction as a part of complex therapy

3. Rivaroxaban + acetylsalicylic acid after autovenous bypass and/or as additional antiplatelet therapy

4. Antiplatelet agents/cilostazol/aducil for chronic arterial obstruction II A–B

5. Thrombolytics

6. NSAIDs for pain syndrome

7. Statins for all patients with chronic arterial obstruction and diabetic neuroosteoarthropathy

8. Tizanidine/gabapentin for seizure disorder

5. Local therapy design

Detersion of wound defect and creating a "platform" for its closure:

5.1 On inpatient basis

1. Hydrosurgical ultrasound (cavitation) treatment of tissue defects.

5.2 On outpatient basis

1. Chemical necrectomy (patent for invention No. 2549459 of 30.03.2015. ROSPATENT FGU FIPS RF)

2. Mechanical necrectomy

3. Interactive bandages

Closure of tissue defects:

- Implantation of xenoplastic biomaterial as part of complex treatment (patent for invention No. 2423118 of 10.06.2011 ROSPATENT FGU FIPS RF and patent for invention No. 2549459 of 30.03.2015 ROSPATENT FGU FIPS RF)

- Combined application of synthetic complex bioplastic materials (patent for invention No. 2619257 of 12.05.2017 ROSPATENT FGU FIPS RF)

- Combination of application of bioplastic collagen material and introduction of autologous growth factors into the wound defect (patent for invention No. 2679449 of 11.02.2019 ROSPATENT FGU FIPS RF)

- Administration of autologous growth factors into tissue defects after autodermoplasty with free split skin grafts.

When carrying out drug build-up and prescriptions for patients with DFS, the antiplatelet agents are the largest group of drugs. It includes a number of various drugs with different application points.

We are primarily interested in cilostazol as a selective phosphodiesterase 3 inhibitor with a three-way effect: vasodilatory, antiplatelet and antithrombotic, with inhibition of phosphodiesterase 3 and, consequently, an increase in the intracellular content of cAMP. It also affects the level of matrix metalloproteases in wound defects, which is important in patients with diabetes mellitus [9].

Therefore, we carried out a molecular study of the mechanisms of action of cilostazol on certain families of phosphodiesterases with the aim of studying the effect of cilostazol on the isoforms of phosphodiesterase three targets and phosphodiesterase 5 using a molecular model; the results of molecular modeling are to be used to predict potential clinical effects when cilostazol administration [10].

The study of phosphodiesterase inhibition was performed using molecular docking methods. Docking was performed using Maestro Schrodinger Inc. software [11]. The structure of all proteins was taken from the Protein Data Bank (PDB): 7L27-PDE3IA, 1JOS-PDE3B, 4MD6-phosphodiesterase 5. The structures of the ligands, that is, cilostazol and vardenafil, were taken from the PubChem database. Glide Docking SP mode was used to determine the best ligand pose in the phosphodiesterase-ligand supramolecular complex with the function of minimum energy evaluation. Each phosphodiesterase molecule was prepared before docking using the Protein Preparation Wizard module. The optimization of the ligand geometry was performed using the MMF4 force field in the GROMACS molecular dynamics software package [12]. The active center of the enzymes was considered to be rigid. Visualization of the results was performed using the Ligand Interaction function in the Maestro module. The inhibition constant (Ki) was obtained from the binding energy (ΔG) using the formula: Ki = exp. (ΔG/RT), where R is the universal gas constant ($1{,}985 \times 10^{-3}$ kcal mol^{-1} K^{-1}) and T is the temperature (298,15 K) [11].

The figures show diagrams comparing the binding energy (ΔG) of cilostazol and two isoforms of phosphodiesterase 3A and phosphodiesterase 3B (**Figure 1**) and the binding energies (ΔG) of cilostazol with phosphodiesterase V against vardenafil—a classical phosphodiesterase 5 selective inhibitor (**Figure 2**).

Following the binding energy assessment, we analyzed key non-covalent interactions of cilostazol, vardenafil with phosphodiesterase 5, and cilostazol with phosphodiesterase 3A and phosphodiesterase 3B, respectively.

The most important interactions are the following (**Figure 3**): 1. The coordination complex between the magnesium ion in the active center of the enzyme and the oxygen atom of the quinolinone group. 2. The hydrogen bond between the nitrogen atom of the quinolinone group and ASP950. 3. π-π stacking interactions between TYR751 and the phenolic ring of the quinoline group.

The most important interactions are the following (**Figure 4**): 1. Hydrogen bonding between GLN 988 and the oxygen and nitrogen atoms of the quinoline group. 2. π-π stacking interactions between PHE991 and the phenol ring of the quinoline group.

The most important interactions are the following (**Figure 5**): 1. Hydrogen bond between GLN 775 and the oxygen atom of the quinoline group. 2. π-π stacking interactions between PHE820 and the phenol ring of the quinoline group.

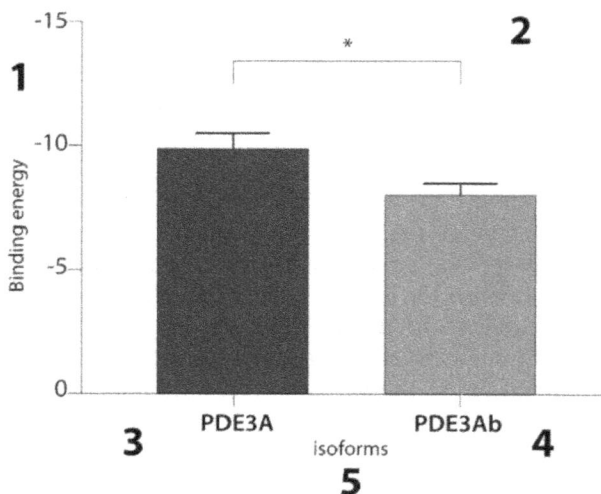

Figure 1.
*Comparison of the binding energy (ΔG) of cilostazol with phosphodiesterase 3A ($-9{,}9 \pm 0{,}455$ kcal/mol) and phosphodiesterase 3B ($-8{,}1 \pm 0{,}324$ kcal/mol). *p < 0,05: 1—binding energy; 2—binding energy of cilostazol with PDE3 isoforms; 3—PDE 3A; 4—PDE 3B; 5—isoforms.*

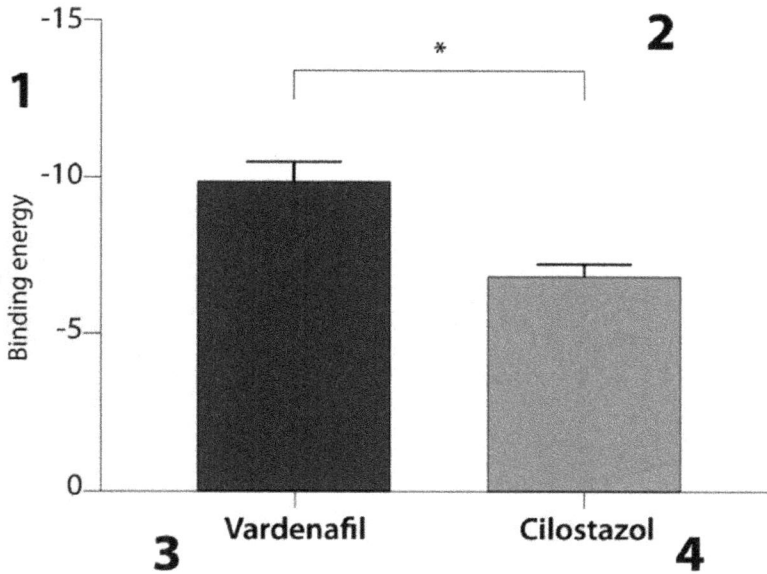

Figure 2.
*Comparison of the binding energy (ΔG) of cilostazol (−6,8 ± 0,32 kcal/mol) and vardenafil (−10,1 ± 0,4 kcal/mol) with phosphodiesterase 5. *p < 0,05: 1—binding energy; 2—binding energy of cilostazol with PDE5 in comparison with vardenafil; 3—vardenafil; 4—cilostazol.*

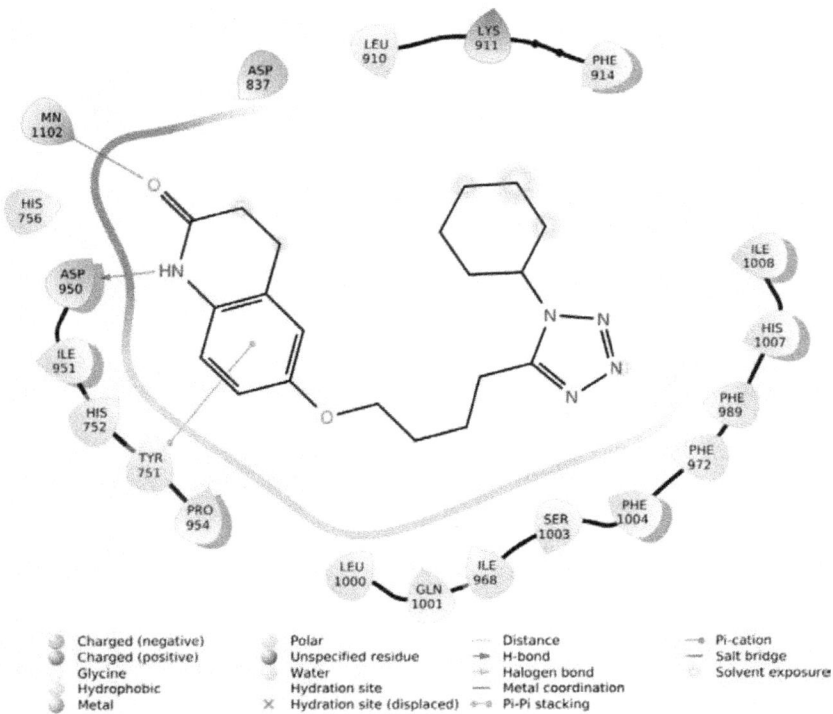

Figure 3.
Key molecular interactions between cilostazol and phosphodiesterase 3A.

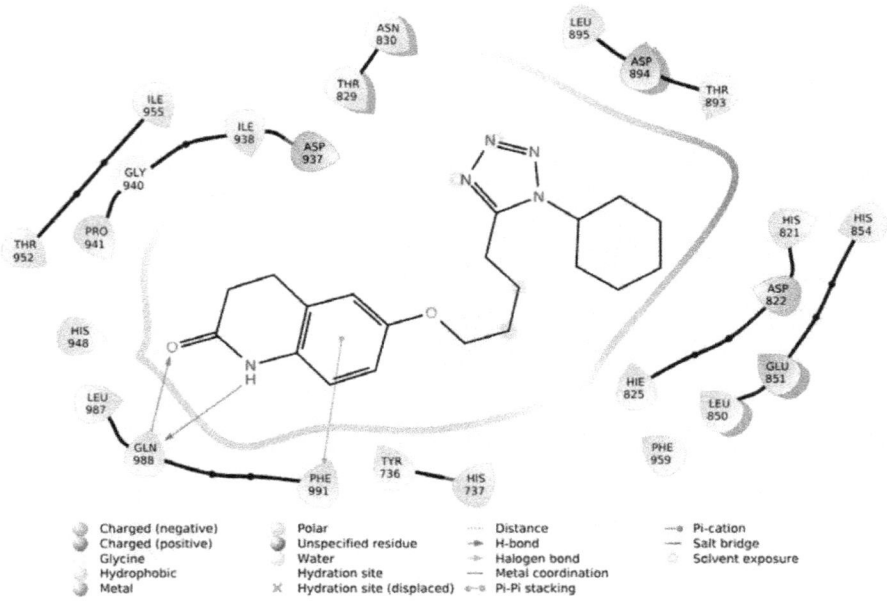

Figure 4.
Key molecular interactions between cilostazol and phosphodiesterase 3B.

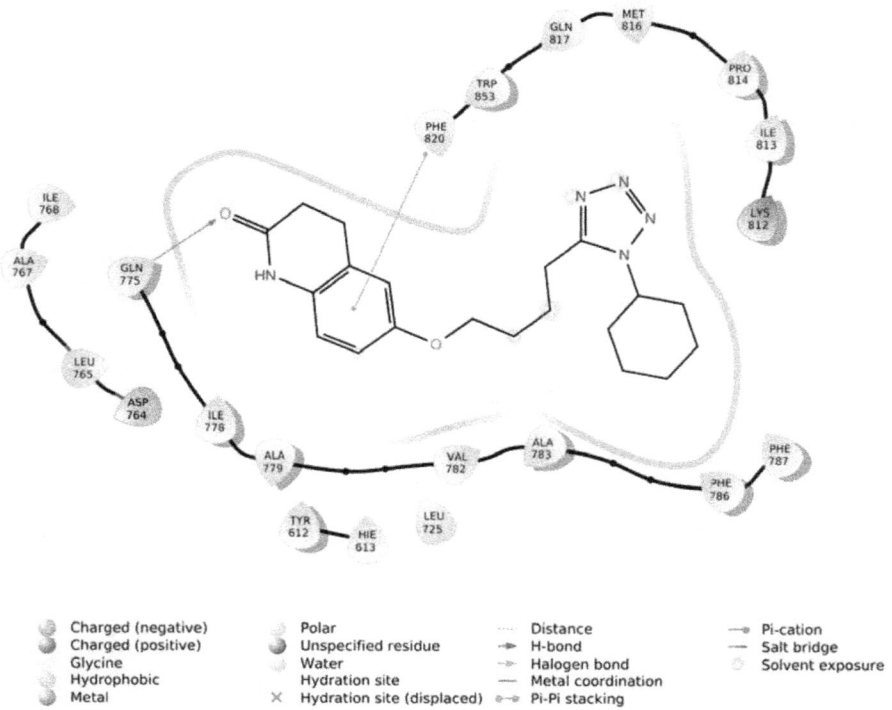

Figure 5.
Key molecular interactions between cilostazol and phosphodiesterase 5.

From The analysis of cilostazol interactions with various active phosphodiesterases centers demonstrates that the quinoline fragment of the cilostazol molecule is key for all of the above-mentioned protein-ligand interactions. The coordination bond of cilostazol with the magnesium atom in phosphodiesterase 3A explains the higher affinity of cilostazol for this form of phosphodiesterase 3. Moreover, the data obtained for the inhibition constant (Ki) of phosphodiesterase 3A and phosphodiesterase 3B (**Table 1**) coincide with those confirmed experimentally, which can serve as a criterion for the correctness of the docking performed and the results evaluation [13]. The calculated inhibition constants (Ki) of phosphodiesterase 5 for cilostazol and vardenafil are shown in **Table 2**.

According to data obtained, cilostazol inhibits the isoform of phosphodiesterase 3A significantly more strongly (Ki = 54 nM) than of phosphodiesterase 3B (Ki = 1,13 μM). This explains the low incidence of side effects from phosphodiesterase 3B inhibition when using cilostazol in clinical practice. However, we cannot help but note that phosphodiesterase 3B is an attractive target for diabetes mellitus treatment, obesity and other metabolic syndrome components. An important link in the pathogenesis of obesity, insulin resistance and metabolic syndrome is inflammation in white adipose tissue, including infiltration and further expansion of macrophages. The key event required for the inflammation development in adipose tissue is the activation of inflammasomes within adipocytes, which subsequently leads to increased caspase-1 levels and IL1β processing, contributing to the occurrence of many metabolic disorders that direct adipocytes to an insulin-resistant phenotype and promote the inflammation development. Inhibition of phosphodiesterase 3B in white adipose tissue prevents activation of inflammasomes by reducing the expression of various proinflammatory genes such as NLRP3, caspase-1, ASC, AIM2, TNFα, IL1β and others [14]. Therefore, the ability of cilostazol, used as a monodrug, to inhibit not only phosphodiesterase 3A, but also phosphodiesterase 3B provides a multifactorial effect on various pathogenesis pathways associated with the phosphodiesterase 3 family in metabolic syndrome, diabetes mellitus, peripheral arterial obliterating disease and obesity.

Cilostazol can also inhibit phosphodiesterase 5 in therapeutic doses (Ki = 10 μM). Cilostazol is thus not a strict inhibitor of the phosphodiesterase 3 family only. It was reliably established that PDE 5 inhibitors have certain prospects in diabetic polyneuropathy treatment and, consequently, diabetic foot syndrome. Thus, in a

Cilostazol	Ki (inhibition constant)
Phosphodiesterase 3A	54 nM
Phosphodiesterase 3B	1,13 μM

Table 1.
Calculated constant of phosphodiesterase 3A and phosphodiesterase 3B inhibition by cilostazol.

Phosphodiesterase 5	Ki (inhibition constant)
Vardenafil	19,7 nM
Cilostazol	10 μM

Table 2.
Calculated constant of phosphodiesterase 5 inhibition by vardenafil and cilostazol.

study by Lei Wang it was found that long-term treatment of mice with diabetes with a phosphodiesterase 5 inhibitor (Tadalafil) significantly increases axonal growth and sciatic nerve myelination, and thus increases conduction velocity and sensory functions [15]. Therefore, the ability of cilostazol to inhibit phosphodiesterase 5 will have an additional therapeutic effect in the treatment of intermittent claudication, diabetes mellitus and its complications, especially neuropathy.

Thus, it was established and predicted potential therapeutic effects of cilostazol application, associated with new molecular data affinity for the phosphodiesterase 3 and phosphodiesterase 5 families, in the complex treatment of diabetic foot syndrome.

Conflict of interests

The author declare no conflict of interest.

Author details

Koreyba Konstantin Aleksandrovich
Department of Surgical Diseases, Kazan State Medical University, Ministry of Health of the Russian Federation, Kazan, Russia

*Address all correspondence to: korejba_k@mail.ru

IntechOpen

References

[1] International Diabetes Federation. IDF Diabetes Atlas. 10th ed. Brussels, Belgium: International Diabetes Federation; 2021

[2] Ozougwu JC, Obimba KC, Belonwu CD, Unakalamba CB. The pathogenesis and pathophysiology of type 1 and 2 diabetes mellitus. Journal of Physiology and Pathophysiology. 2013;**4**(4):46-57

[3] Stupin VA, Silina EV, Koreyba KA, Goryunov SV. Diabetic Foot Syndrome: Epidemiology, Pathophysiology, Diagnostics and Treatment. Moscow: Litterra; 2019. 198 p.: tab., color ill.; 22 cm; ISBN 978-5-4235-0324-6

[4] Bova AA, Koroleva AA, Zhuravkov YL. Effect of drugs on bone tissue. Military Medicine. 2009;**2**:27-30

[5] Bensman VM. Surgery of Purulent-Necrotic Complications of the Diabetic Foot [Text]: A Manual for Doctors. Ministry of Health of the Russian Federation, State Budgetary Educational Institution of Higher Professional Education "Kuban State Medical University", National Healthcare Institution of Higher Professional Education "Kuban Medical Institute", State Healthcare Institution "Krasnodar Regional Clinical Hospital No. 1 named after prof. S. V. Ochapovsky". 2nd revised and additional ed. Moscow: Medpraktika-M; 2015. 495 p.: ill., tab., color ill.: 21 cm; ISBN 978-5-98803-326-4

[6] Barengolts EI, Berman M, Kukreja SC, Kouznetsova T, Lin C, Chomka EV. Osteoporosis and coronary atherosclerosis in asymptomatic postmenopausal women. Calcified Tissue International. 1998;**62**(3):209-213. DOI: 10.1007/s002239900419

[7] Parhami F, Garfinkel A, Demer LL. Role of lipids in osteoporosis. Arteriosclerosis, Thrombosis, and Vascular Biology: Journal of the American Heart Association. 2000;**20**:2346-2348. Available from: https://api.semanticscholar.org/CorpusID:12551993

[8] Russell RGG, Rogers MJ, Frith JC, Luckman SP, Coxon FP, Benford HL, et al. The pharmacology of bisphosphonates and new insights into their mechanisms of action. Journal of Bone and Mineral Research. 1999;**14**(S2):53-65. DOI: 10.1002/jbmr.5650140212

[9] de Franciscis S et al. Cilostazol prevents foot ulcers in diabetic patients with peripheral vascular disease. International Wound Journal. 2015;**12**(3):250-253

[10] Koreyba KA, Stupin VA, Silina EV, Syuzev KN, Serebryakova OA. Molecular study of mecha nisms of action of cilostazol on certain families of phosphodiesterases. Angiology and Vascular Surgery. 2022;**28**(1):22-28. DOI: 10.33029/1027-6661-2022-28-1-22-28. (in Russian)

[11] Friesner RA, Murphy RB, Repasky MP, et al. Extra precision glide: Docking and scoring incorporating a model of hydrophobic enclosure for protein-ligand complexes. Journal of Medicinal Chemistry. 2006;**49**(21):6177-6196. DOI: 10.1021/jm051256o

[12] Berendsen HJC, van der Spoel D, van Drunen R. GROMACS: A message-passing7arallel molecular dynamics implementation. Computer Physics Communications. 1995;**91**:43-56. DOI: 10.1016/0010-4655(95)00042-E

[13] Atkins PW, De PJ. Atkins' Physical Chemistry. Oxford: Oxford University Press; 2006

[14] Ahmad F, Chung YW, Tang Y, et al. Phosphodiesterase 3B (PDE3B) regulates NLRP3 inflammasome in adipose tissue. Scientific Reports. 2016;**6**:28056. DOI: 10.1038/srep28056

[15] Wang L, Chopp M, Zhang ZG. PDE5 inhibitors promote recovery of peripheral neuropathy in diabetic mice. Neural Regeneration Research. 2017;**12**(2):218-219. DOI: 10.4103/1673-5374.200804

Chapter 3

Molecular Imaging Methods in Evaluation of Diabetic Foot

Leszek Królicki, Julia Stępień-Dziekan, Konrad Giełdowski and Bartosz Sawicki

Abstract

Clinical exams and blood tests are essential tools for healthcare providers evaluating patients with suspected osteomyelitis, but they are often inadequate for a definitive diagnosis. Therefore, imaging techniques are crucial for diagnosing and, at times, monitoring the complications of diabetic foot. There is still no consensus on the optimal imaging approach for diagnosing both infective and non-infective complications in diabetic foot. The most frequently used advanced imaging techniques include magnetic resonance imaging (MRI) and various nuclear medicine (NM) procedures, such as radiolabelled white blood cell (WBC) scintigraphy and fluorine-18 Fluorodeoxyglucose positron emission tomography/computed tomography ($[^{18}F]$ FDG-PET/CT). Specifically, they should be considered when there is a need to more accurately evaluate the location, extent, or severity of an infection, in order to plan a more personalised treatment and monitor its effectiveness.

Keywords: PET, SPECT, scintigraphy, markers of inflammation, osteomyelitis

1. Introduction

Imaging methods in the assessment of biological processes are based on specific physical phenomena: radiological methods are based on the assessment of differences in the physical density of normal tissues and pathological changes, MRI—on differences in magnetic properties, and ultrasound on differences in the ability to absorb and reflect ultrasound waves. Radioisotope methods require *in vivo* administration of a trace amount of a specific chemical compound, labelled with an appropriate radioisotope (radiopharmaceutical) and measurement of the distribution of radioactivity in the patient's body. This allows for characterisation of the disease process. For this reason, each imaging method has specific limitations, and none of the techniques alone can provide all the relevant indicators of the disease process.

Imaging techniques can be divided into two groups: functional and morphological imaging. Morphological imaging techniques include CT, many MRI protocols and ultrasound. These methods allow for the assessment of disease changes only when pathological processes lead to changes in the structure of the examined organs. However, morphological changes are the final stage of the disease process. Functional disorders are observed much earlier. Therefore, functional imaging techniques,

IntechOpen

especially molecular imaging, are currently a particularly important tool both in understanding pathophysiological processes and in everyday medical diagnostics. Molecular imaging is defined as the non-invasive visualisation, characterisation and measurement of biological processes at the molecular and cellular level in humans and other living systems [1]. This approach can facilitate the non-invasive visualisation of molecular processes such as gene expression and protein synthesis, degradation and interaction *in vivo*.

Molecular imaging techniques include magnetic resonance imaging (MRI) with dedicated sequences and molecular contrast agents, optical imaging (including bioluminescence and immunofluorescence imaging), but above all, nuclear medicine techniques (in particular positron emission tomography [PET]). It is important to note the sensitivity of these imaging methods: the best example is a comparison of the sensitivity of a typical MRI scan and a PET scan. Current MRI machines can only detect a different magnetic signal when the concentration of the chemical substance being examined is greater than 10^{-4} moles, while a PET scan can detect changes in the concentration of a radiopharmaceutical when the difference in its concentration is only 10^{-11} moles.

In medical practice, both methods—morphological and functional—are combined using hybrid imaging techniques (PET/CT, PET/MRI and SPECT/CT): radioisotope examination allows for a more accurate assessment of pathological changes, while CT examination enables better determination of the location of the pathological change and the use of corrective techniques—thanks to which functional images are much more visible (this applies primarily to the correction of the phenomenon of ionising radiation absorption).

The objectives of molecular imaging are:

- to understand the biology of disease processes, including cancer and inflammation,

- to visualise and non-invasively determine the stage of the disease process (active/inactive),

- studying the pharmacokinetics and pharmacodynamics of new targeted therapies,

- determining and predicting the response to new drugs at an early stage of therapy.

2. Clinical problem and pathomechanism of diabetic foot

One of the basic complications of diabetes, alongside damage to the kidney, heart, and retinopathy, is infection of the foot (diabetic foot ulceration; DFU) [2]. The number of patients with this complication will increase due to the obesity epidemic and the ageing population. The population most at risk of developing DFU are men with type 2 diabetes and a low body mass index, long duration of diabetes, diabetic retinopathy, and a history of smoking and hypertension [2]. Foot ulcers are observed in approximately one-quarter of all people with diabetes [3].

The main pathological factors that increase the risk of foot infections in patients with diabetes are diabetic neuropathy, muscle atrophy and Charcot arthropathy [4].

Diabetic neuropathy is defined as a complex polyneuropathy involving damage to peripheral, motor and autonomic neurons [5, 6]. It occurs in 10.9–32.7% of patients with diabetes [7, 8]. Neuropathy results in sensory disturbances that predispose to numerous microtraumas [9]. These injuries can ultimately lead to ulceration and subsequent infection.

Muscle atrophy is caused by motor neuropathy resulting from the loss of myelin fibres [10]. It leads to foot deformities (claw foot, hollow foot, hallux valgus). These biomechanical changes cause gait disturbances and predispose patients with neuropathy to foot ulcers due to increased pressure and shear.

Charcot arthropathy develops in 13% of patients with diabetic neuropathy [11, 12]. This is an inflammatory, potentially destructive foot disease mainly affecting the tarsal and metatarsal joints. Charcot foot may coexist with (or cause) diabetic foot ulcers and may accompany an infectious process [13–15].

An additional factor is autonomic fibre dysfunction in the lower limb, vascular insufficiency (micro- and macrovascular) and immune dysfunction. Autonomic dysfunction causes dilation of blood vessels and excessive warming of the foot. Impaired sweat gland function leads to dry skin and increased susceptibility to microtrauma [16, 17]. Immune dysfunction, in the event of a breach in the protective skin barrier, promotes the development of infection in the wound and vascular disorders limit the migration of phagocytic cells and the delivery of antibiotic therapy. These processes dramatically complicate the treatment of infection.

The infection begins with soft tissue (STI). However, the typical symptoms do not determine the severity of the disease. If the disease process is not stopped, osteomyelitis (OM) occurs, one of the most dangerous complications, as it is associated with a high risk of lower limb amputation, prolonged hospitalisation, high social and financial costs, and increased mortality. Reduced mobility of patients contributes additionally to increased mortality associated with cardiovascular diseases (myocardial infarction, heart failure and stroke) [18–20].

Accurate diagnosis of DFU is a clinical challenge because the main symptoms and signs of infection may be masked (or mimicked) by the presence of peripheral neuropathy or ischaemia, and positive wound culture results may only reflect colonisation of the overlying soft tissues rather than infection. Once a diabetic foot infection has been diagnosed, the severity of the disease must be determined. Three stages of severity have been adopted: mild (involving only a limited area of superficial skin and soft tissues), moderate (more extensive infection, horizontal or vertical) or severe (accompanied by symptoms of a systemic inflammatory response) [21].

3. Diagnostic procedures

The differential diagnosis between osteomyelitis, soft tissue infection and Charcot foot is of key clinical importance, as these three conditions require completely different treatment methods.

The basic diagnostic methods include: a detailed clinical history (especially of any recent but healed wounds or antimicrobial therapy), physical examination (to detect signs of peripheral neuropathy or peripheral arterial disease in the affected foot), blood tests (to check blood sugar levels, routine chemical tests and inflammatory markers) and plain X-rays of the foot and probe-to-bone test (PTB). The results of these methods are often inconclusive. This requires further advanced testing [22].

PTB is a simple clinical test used to assess osteomyelitis in cases of diabetic foot ulcers. It involves inserting a sterile probe into the ulcer and palpating the bone, which indicates a possible bone infection. If the probe reaches the bone, the test is considered positive, suggesting the presence of osteomyelitis. The accuracy of the test may vary depending on the likelihood of osteomyelitis and the clinical situation prior to the test [17, 23]. It must be stressed that PTB is useful but not definitive, especially in the presence of severe neuropathy. A pooled sensitivity and specificity of the PTB test is 87% and 83%, respectively, PPV—98% and NPV—72%. The diagnostic accuracy can be improved by combining ESR and PTB. If either test is positive, the sensitivity and specificity amount to 96% and 65.7%, respectively. When the result of the PTB test is combined with that of plain X-rays, the sensitivity increases to 88.6%, but the specificity falls to 66.7% [24].

The golden standard for the final diagnosis of OM is still a bone biopsy. The test provides histological and microbiological information [25]. It also allows for determining the type of bacteria responsible for the inflammation and their sensitivity to various antibiotics. This procedure is, however, invasive and not always feasible, but it is possible to establish a bacterial microbiota based on the culture of deep soft tissue that is in direct contact with the bone. A good correlation has been shown between the bacterial microbiota obtained from a bone biopsy and the deep tissues of the ulcer. Therefore, a bone biopsy can be replaced by a procedure confirming bone inflammation and a bacterial microbiota from the deep tissues of the ulcer.

X-ray examination plays a crucial role in diagnosing and managing diabetic foot complications, particularly osteomyelitis and other bony issues. It is a readily available and relatively inexpensive imaging technique that can help detect fractures, joint dislocations, and infection. However, X-rays may not be sensitive enough to detect early stages of osteomyelitis, and serial radiographs may be needed for more definitive diagnosis [26]. X-ray sensitivity in diagnosing diabetic foot osteomyelitis is between 43% and 75% and specificity is between 75% and 83% [27]. X-rays can also help identify other diabetic foot complications, such as Charcot osteoarthropathy, gout, and vascular calcifications [28].

The most commonly used advanced imaging method is magnetic resonance imaging (MRI). MRI has a high potential for diagnosing deep abscesses, tendon ruptures, and septic exudate in joint cavities. Symptomatic MRI findings of inflammation include: decreased marrow signal intensity on T1-w images, increased marrow signal intensity on fluid-sensitive sequences and post-contrast enhancement [29]. An MRI scan may show symptoms of Charcot osteoarthropathy already in a very early stage, as well as bone and cartilage changes, bone marrow oedema, hidden fractures, and joint effusion. According to meta-analyses, MRI is the best diagnostic tool in diabetic foot imaging [30, 31]. For MRI, the overall accuracy is 84%. Some data suggested that MRI is more cost-effective, with the exception of patients with initially low disease probability [32]. On the other hand, MRI has many limitations: MRI may not always accurately differentiate between osteomyelitis and other conditions like Charcot neuroarthropathy or soft tissue inflammation (especially in the presence of oedema or non-enhancing tissue). Additionally, MRI's effectiveness can vary across different foot regions and may be affected by vascular issues, leading to false positives or negatives. MRI sensitivity (correctly identifying osteomyelitis) is high, but specificity (correctly identifying the absence of osteomyelitis) can be lower, especially in the tarsal bones. Decreased blood flow (ischaemia) in the diabetic foot can lead to false-negative MRI results, where osteomyelitis is present but not detected. Conversely, conditions with increased blood flow (hyperemia) can cause false-positive results, suggesting osteomyelitis when it is not present [33]. Other limitations of MRI examination include the presence of metal implants, examination time, and availability.

4. Radioisotopic procedures

Various nuclear medicine procedures play an important role in characterising the disease process. The mechanisms of accumulation of selected radiopharmaceuticals in the inflammatory focus are very different. For this reason, individual procedures demonstrate different diagnostic accuracy.

4.1 Three-phase bone scintigraphy

This method typically employs diphosphonates tagged with Technetium-99 m (^{99m}Tc), which attach to the hydroxyapatite crystals within the bone. The level of tracer uptake is influenced by blood circulation, the bone remodelling rate (osteoblastic activity), and the presence of calcium deposits [34].

For imaging of osteomyelitis, typically a three-phase imaging protocol is used, and sometimes a four-phase approach is applied. The angiographic phase, also known as the blood flow phase, is captured immediately after tracer administration for about 60 seconds. The soft tissue or blood pool phase images are taken 5–10 minutes later. The bone phase, or delayed images, are obtained 3–4 hours post-injection. Optimal imaging results are achieved when patients are well hydrated, which helps increase the contrast between the target area and background bone activity. If greater specificity is required, a fourth phase is performed 24 hours after tracer injection [35].

A normal bone scan across all phases (arterial, venous, and bone) effectively excludes bone infection because of its high sensitivity. However, the technique suffers from low specificity, as it often produces false-positive results caused by factors such as bone remodelling, injuries, arthritis, recent surgical procedures, or Charcot arthropathy, whether or not an infection is present. Conducting SPECT/CT during the delayed phase enables precise anatomical identification of the bone-forming process, thereby enhancing the test's accuracy (**Figure 1**).

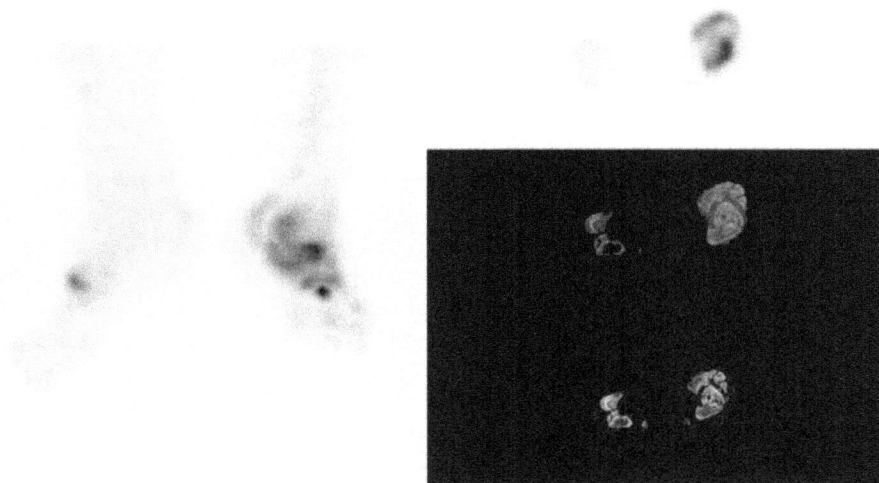

Figure 1.
Increased tracer uptake within the tarsal bones of the left foot in three-phase bone scintigraphy after administration of [^{99m}Tc]Tc-MDP by a hybrid SPECT/CT method in the third phase of the examination – an image typical of Charcot foot. Left: maximum intensity projection (MIP) targeting the foot. Right: transverse views (from top): functional (SPECT), fusion (SPECT/CT) and structural (CT) images.

The primary limitation of planar nuclear medicine imaging is its low spatial resolution and absence of clear anatomical reference points, which poses a particular challenge in the foot due to the small size and close proximity of the bones. Uptake seen in soft tissues on planar images can overlap with the underlying bone, and vice versa, potentially causing misinterpretation of the scan and leading to incorrect treatment decisions. For this reason, as mentioned earlier, using hybrid imaging techniques is essential to enhance the diagnostic accuracy of planar scans [36].

No significant difference in the amputation rate for patients with confirmatory, indeterminate, or nonconfirmatory three-phase bone scans for osteomyelitis was found. Therefore, the authors conclude that the ultimate treatment decision should be based on clinical indicators of the presence of uncontrolled infection or gangrene rather than on bone scan findings [37].

Summarising, the three-phase bone scan is now primarily limited to ruling out infection due to its strong negative predictive value, with little other clinical use remaining [38, 39].

4.2 Scintigraphy with labelled leukocytes

Scintigraphy with labelled leukocytes is an imaging method widely used in the diagnosis of inflammation. It involves labelling white blood cells and assessing their distribution in the body using a gamma-camera scan. This method uses the phenomenon of chemotaxis – it assumes that labelled leukocytes retain the ability to chemotaxis and accumulate in infectious foci. Acquisition is usually performed in two parts, at 4 and 24 hours after administration of the radiolabelled leukocytes, or in three parts: at 30 minutes and at 3 and 20 hours, both with registration of planar images and SPECT/CT [40].

Several radiopharmaceuticals of choice are used to label leukocytes, and can be divided into two groups depending on the method of labelling: *in vivo* (using ^{99m}Tc-labelled antibodies) and *in vitro* (using [^{111}In]In-oxide or [^{99m}Tc]Tc-HMPAO).

The *in vivo* method involves direct intravenous administration of ^{99m}Tc-labelled antibodies that specifically bind to the surface antigen of granulocytes migrating to inflammatory foci. Mouse monoclonal antibodies (e.g., besilesomab, sulesomab, and fanolesomab) or modified human IgG immunoglobulin are used. These will include anti-NCA90-Fab, murine MoAb IgG that is cross-reactive to antigen 95 on neutrophils, anti-CD15 antigen and DPC-11870 that targets the leukotriene B4 receptors of granulocytes. In the case of antibodies of mouse origin, the risk of an immune reaction with the production of anti-mouse antibodies (HAMA) must be taken into account [36]. Therefore, before administering the radiopharmaceutical, a test for HAMA should be performed, and a history of previous similar reactions should be taken or the patient is advised not to repeat the test with this preparation in the future. However, many comparative analyses do not include testing with anti-granulocyte antibodies because of their limited use in the diagnosis of diabetic foot [41]. This may be due to the presence of a large mass of labelled molecules, limiting their diffusion into inflammatory lesions in this area of the body [36]. Some authors advocate performing dual scintigraphy: three-phase bone scintigraphy and granulocyte-radiolabelled scintigraphy, with the assumption that a positive result of both scans means osteitis, and that positive granulocyte scanning only indicates soft-tissue involvement [42]. Hybrid SPECT/CT scanning does not significantly contribute to the evaluation of patients with negative scan results [43]. As the labelled leukocytes accumulate in uninfected neuropathic joints, bone marrow scintigraphy may be needed to determine whether infection is present [44].

In vitro methods require caution to avoid damaging leukocytes and to follow special aseptic rules. In addition, the preparation procedure is complicated and time-consuming [45]. Nowadays, $[^{99m}Tc]$Tc-HMPAO is more commonly used because of obtaining better image quality, easier availability and less radiation exposure than after using $[^{111}In]$In-oxide.

Scintigraphy with labelled leukocytes has also found its way into the diagnosis of diabetic foot infections. Like other advanced imaging modalities, it is designed to determine the risk of an STI and pinpoint its location in order to accurately biopsy and microbiologically test for appropriate treatment. In addition, it is mostly used in assessing the extent of inflammatory lesions and in differentiating STI, OM and Charcot osteoarthropathy and the effectiveness of treatment [38, 45]. It is used when other methods fail to clearly determine its presence, including laboratory markers (ESR, CRP) and radiography, and MRI, which is usually the first choice in such a situation, fails to determine the presence of inflammatory lesions due to its lower specificity than WBC scintigraphy, and when it is unavailable or contraindicated [40].

As mentioned earlier, scintigraphy images with labelled leukocytes are specific for different types of complications of diabetic foot infection. In soft tissue infection, increased focal or diffuse activity is seen in early images, which stabilises or decreases in late images. SPECT/CT images show increased accumulation in soft tissues [36]. In osteomyelitis, increasing focal activity is seen in late images (**Figure 2**), compared to images recorded in early images, while focal accumulation in bone tissue is seen in SPECT/CT images. Charcot osteoarthropathy is characterised by diffuse activity in late images and less or stable activity compared to early images. On SPECT/CT, tracer accumulation correlates with bone destruction [36]. However, bone marrow expansion secondary to chronic inflammation must be taken into account, lowering the specificity of this method. To this end, bone marrow scintigraphy (BMS) using nanocolloids is suggested. In case of concordance, that is, both positive results, the similarity of the diagnosis of Charcot disease increases, while with a positive white blood cell scintigraphy and a negative result with nanocolloid, osteomyelitis can be diagnosed [36, 45]. The need for expanded diagnosis may be due to the location of the lesions, as significantly higher sensitivity and specificity have been demonstrated in

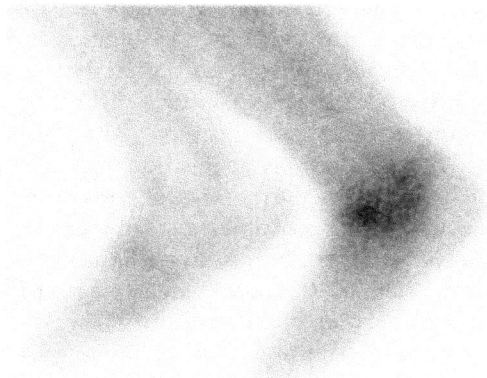

Figure 2.
Features of inflammation in the tarsal bones of the left foot, as well as the forefoot and tarsal region of the right foot on scintigraphy with labelled leukocytes. Planar image in lateral projection.

the forefoot than in the midfoot or hindfoot, which is related to the presence of physiological tracer uptake in the expanded bone marrow of the posterior bony structures of the foot [36, 40].

Importantly, the effect of antibiotic treatment on the sensitivity of leukocyte-labelled scintigraphy, which is also used to assess the effectiveness of treatment, has not been clearly demonstrated. According to the recommendations, such patients should not be excluded if the test needs to be performed. However, too much concern on the part of some experts about obtaining false-negative results has resulted in the common practice of performing the test 2 weeks after cessation of therapy [36].

4.3 PET examination

Positron emission tomography (PET) with 18-fluorodeoxyglucose ($[^{18}F]FDG$) is a nuclear medicine examination that relies on detecting sites of abnormally increased glucose metabolism within the patient's body. This technique involves the intravenous administration of modified glucose particles labelled with radioactive fluorine-18. In macrophages and phagocytic cells, $[^{18}F]FDG$ is transported *via* d-glucose transporter and is phosphorylated by hexokinase resulting in $[^{18}F]FDG$-6 phosphate [46–48]. The high tissue radioactivity after administration of $[^{18}F]FDG$ corresponds to increased glucose uptake and consumption, which is the main source of energy for chemotaxis and phagocytosis [49–51]. In the acute phase of inflammation, a high $[^{18}F]FDG$ uptake is detected in neutrophils, while in the chronic phase the uptake of the tracer is seen in macrophages and polymorphonuclear leukocytes. The examination is commonly performed as a hybrid imaging incorporating computed tomography (CT) for attenuation correction and better localisation of the detected pathologies.

In diabetic patients, the main indication for $[^{18}F]FDG$-PET examination is the diagnosis of diabetic foot osteomyelitis, especially in patients with soft tissue ulcers accompanied by high suspicion of the disease affecting bone structure due to the results of the clinical examination, probe-to-bone test and radiographs [52]. Recent meta-analyses show that $[^{18}F]FDG$-PET imaging has a high sensitivity of about 84%, and an even higher specificity of about 93% for detecting osteomyelitis [53], meaning the examination has a similar sensitivity but higher specificity than MRI. The acquisition field of view is usually limited to the feet, except in patients at risk of sepsis. This makes it one of the shortest imaging procedures performed in this indication. Footholders are commonly used to prevent unnecessary movements during the examination. The site of inflammation is characterised by an increased focal or diffuse uptake localised to the bone or extending from an adjacent soft tissue ulcer [54]. The $[^{18}F]FDG$-PET examination should be accompanied by a CT thin slice acquisition reconstructed with bone matrix in all orthogonal planes, to verify the presence of any erosions or osseous destruction. It is also useful for excluding other probable causes of increased $[^{18}F]FDG$ uptake, such as fractures, metastases, or degenerative diseases. The accurate registration of $[^{18}F]$ FDG-PET images is crucial in cases of intense soft tissue uptake and suspected blooming into the bone, in which the manipulation of the intensity of the window is required to properly define the epicentre of the lesion and evaluate for bone involvement. There is also a possibility for replacing CT with MRI, which could theoretically positively impact the examination's accuracy, yet the data for it is currently very limited [35].

Increased $[^{18}F]FDG$ uptake can also be observed in other types of infections associated with diabetic foot. In patients with soft tissue infection, the uptake is either focal or diffuse and restricted only to soft tissues (**Figure 3**) [54]. Recent studies show that in these cases, the PET examination has a high specificity, but its sensitivity is lower than that of the WBC-labelled SPECT/CT [41]. There are also indications that the [^{18}F] FDG-PET could be used for differentiation between osteomyelitis and diabetic foot neuropathic-osteoarthropathy (Charcot), especially in patients with mid- and hindfoot ulcers. In patients with Charcot, the diffuse radiotracer uptake is localised to the joints. This, however, requires further verification, as the data for this topic is still scarce.

It is important to note that the assessment of [^{18}F]FDG-PET in the cases of diabetic foot infection is mostly qualitative. A semi-quantitative approach incorporating SUVmax values was attempted in the past, with singular studies showing higher values in patients with osteomyelitis compared to soft tissue infection, Charcot, or uncomplicated diabetic foot [36]. Further analyses, however, did not confirm this data and no definite cutoff values could be established.

Despite many positive qualities of [^{18}F]FDG-PET, it also has a few downsides. First of all, it does not allow for differentiation between infection and sterile inflammation. Furthermore, as the qualitatively assessed examination, its sensitivity relies on personal experience [36]. It is also highly impacted by serum insulin and glucose concentration, with high latter levels interfering with the [^{18}F]FDG uptake [54]. Therefore, it can be problematic to perform the examination in patients with poorly controlled diabetes. Imaging should be acquired with the lowest possible serum glucose level. In patients treated with insulin, it needs to be scheduled in consideration of the time of breakfast consumption, to preserve the necessary time between the insulin injection, the meal, and the examination. Another important factor is antibiotic therapy, which can impact the [^{18}F]FDG uptake patterns. The examination should preferably be performed before the antibiotic treatment, but at the same time, it should not be the cause for the delay in therapy. The impact of the antibiotics on the results of [^{18}F]FDG-PET could be potentially used to assess the effectiveness of the medication, yet there is not enough data to verify its usefulness in this indication. Another group of medications that could impact the imaging is glucocorticosteroids. If the patient is to receive such medication, the examination should

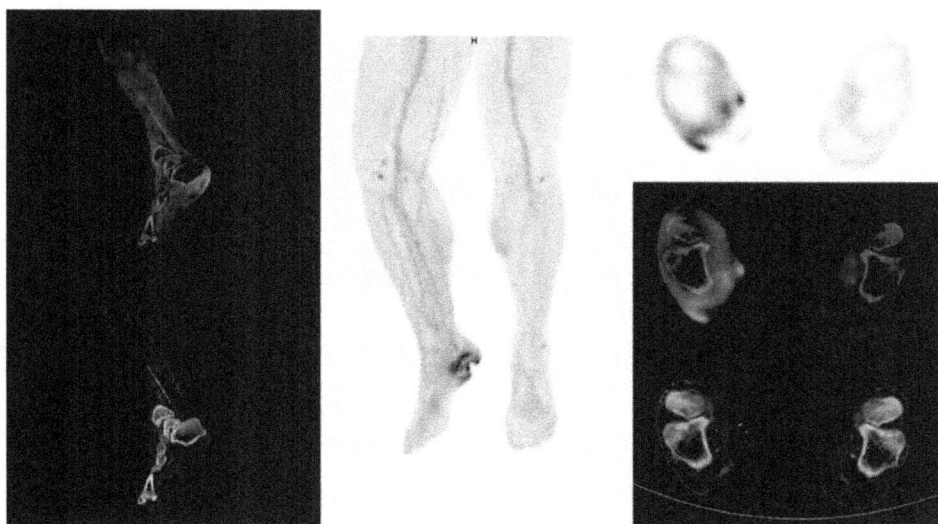

Figure 3.
Increased, diffuse tracer uptake in the area of the right heel with extensive soft tissue loss visible, without bone involvement in [^{18}F]FDG-PET/CT—an image typical of soft tissue infection. Left: sagittal view: fusion image (PET/CT)—above, structural image (CT)—below. Middle: maximum intensity projection (MIP). Right: transverse views (from top): functional (PET), fusion (PET/CT) and structural (CT) images.

be performed within 3 days from the start of the therapy. Longer treatment with steroids substantially decreases the [18F]FDG uptake and the sensitivity of the examination.

4.4 Other radiopharmaceuticals

4.4.1 [67Ga]Ga-citrate

Gallium citrate ([67Ga]Ga-citrate) is the oldest radiopharmaceutical used in the diagnosis of infections; it was employed for over 30 years. After intravenous (i.v.) administration, it binds primarily to transferrin and to other iron-binding proteins such as lactoferrin, ferritin, and bacterial siderophores. Thereafter, it concentrates in lysosomes and is bound to a soluble intracellular protein in inflammation foci as well primary and metastatic tumours, allowing their scintigraphic localisation. [67Ga]Ga-citrate is sensitive for imaging acute infection, chronic infection, and inflammation. [67Ga]Ga-citrate scintigraphy cannot differentiate between tumour and acute inflammation. Nowadays, it is rarely used and is being replaced by other labelled radiopharmaceuticals, mainly 99mTc, due to better image quality, lower radiation exposure for the patient, and a simplified examination protocol. [67Ga]Ga-citrate examination has a high specificity, but the accuracy rate is only 70% [54–56].

4.4.2 [99mTc]Tc-nanocolloid

Nanocolloid is a human albumin. When administered subcutaneously, it is used for lymphoscintigraphy, whereas when administered intravenously, it is used for bone marrow scintigraphy and the diagnosis of inflammatory conditions. Labelled nanocolloid accumulates physiologically in the bone marrow as well as in the reticuloendothelial system of the liver and spleen. In inflammatory foci, it accumulates non-specifically due to increased vascular permeability at the site of inflammation [57].

4.4.3 Radiolabelled antibiotics

In an attempt to differentiate bacterial infection and sterile inflammation, antibiotics that penetrate bacterial cell wall and kill microorganisms by various mechanisms were radiolabelled and evaluated [58, 59]. The most commonly used among them to image infection is ciprofloxacin (Infecton). Ciprofloxacin is a synthetic broad-spectrum fluoroquinolone antibiotic that binds to bacterial DNA gyrase and inhibits DNA synthesis [60, 61]. Ciprofloxacin can be labelled with 99mTc, 68Ga and 18F.

Clinical studies of [99mTc]Tc-Infecton have concluded that this radiopharmaceutical can be used for imaging tuberculosis, osteomyelitis, orthopaedic prosthesis, spinal infection, abdominal infections, and infection in immunosuppressed patients [62, 63]. Other promising antibiotics have been evaluated [58, 59].

4.4.4 Amino acids

The possibility of using amino acids as radiopharmaceuticals in the diagnosis of inflammation has also been investigated. The use of D-stereoisomers of amino acids seems to be particularly interesting because they occur in the cell walls of bacteria but are not present in humans. Therefore, these amino acid isoforms are promising pathogen-specific imaging targets [64, 65].

5. Conclusions

Diagnostics and treatment of complications related to the course of diabetes are one of the important clinical problems. A particularly difficult task is the prevention and treatment of diabetic foot syndrome. A prerequisite for proper treatment is accurate identification and differentiation of the different types of DFU. The basic diagnostic tools are imaging methods. However, no imaging method can present all important aspects of the disease process. The use of multimodal imaging and a multidisciplinary approach is mandatory in order to plan the most appropriate therapeutic strategy for an individual patient.

According to current clinical guidelines, including the EANM guideline [54], it should be assumed that in patients with a foot wound, a positive PTB test and the X-ray, OM should be diagnosed without the need for further imaging. However, advanced imaging using MRI, WBC SPECT/CT, or [^{18}F]FDG-PET/CT may be necessary if the X-ray result is normal and the laboratory tests indicate an inflammatory process. Additional tests are also necessary for patients in whom the exact location, extent, or severity of the infection needs to be determined to plan more tailored treatment and monitor its effectiveness. These tests are also indicated to monitor the therapy and determine whether the infection has resolved. In the case of suspected STI, WBC, MRI, and [^{18}F]FDG-PET/CT have comparable accuracy. Performing one of these tests is especially recommended if the MRI image is equivocal. MRI is the method of choice in the diagnosis of Charcot neuro-osteoarthropathy. However, it does not allow for the exclusion of the inflammatory process in this group of patients. It is believed that the next most sensitive method is WBC SPECT/CT, together with a bone marrow scan. [^{18}F]FDG-PET/CT can be used as an alternative. In most cases, decisions to order imaging tests are best made through multidisciplinary discussion with all specialists involved in the care of these patients. This approach allows for the adaptation of diagnostic and therapeutic strategies to each patient. Larger multicenter studies are still needed to create standardised diagnostic schemes that could be used worldwide (**Table 1**).

	MRI	WBC scan	FDG-PET	Bone scan
Sensitivity	93%	91%	89%	81%
Specificity	75%	92%	92%	28.5%
Limitations	Low specificity metal implants	Complicated preparation of the labelled leucocytes	Lower sensitivity	Low specificity
Accessibility	Moderate	Low	Low	High
Cost	Moderate	Moderate	High	Low
Indication	First method in patients with an equivocal diagnosis of OM based on X-ray	Equivocal results on MRI	Equivocal results on MRI	Ruling out OM

Data of sensitivity and specificity from [38, 54].

Table 1.
Comparison of different molecular imaging procedures in evaluation of diabetic foot.

Author details

Leszek Królicki*, Julia Stępień-Dziekan, Konrad Giełdowski and Bartosz Sawicki
Nuclear Medicine Department, Medical University of Warsaw, Warsaw, Poland

*Address all correspondence to: leszek.krolicki@wum.edu.pl

IntechOpen

References

[1] Pysz MA, Gambhir SS, Willmann JK. Molecular imaging: Current status and emerging strategies. Clinical Radiology. 2010;**65**(7):500-516

[2] Zhang P, Lu J, Jing Y, Tang S, Zhu D, Bi Y. Global epidemiology of diabetic foot ulceration: A systematic review and meta-analysis (dagger). Annals of Medicine. 2017;**49**(2):106-116

[3] Hicks CW, Selvin E. Epidemiology of peripheral neuropathy and lower extremity disease in diabetes. Current Diabetes Reports. 2019;**19**(10):86-99

[4] Kim J. The pathophysiology of diabetic foot: A narrative review. Journal of Yeungnam Medical Science. 2023;**40**(4):328-334

[5] Ponirakis G, Elhadd T, Chinnaiyan S, Dabbous Z, Siddiqui M, Al-Muhannadi H, et al. Prevalence and management of diabetic neuropathy in secondary care in Qatar. Diabetes/Metabolism Research and Reviews. 2020;**36**(4):e3286

[6] Juster-Switlyk K, Smith AG. Updates in diabetic peripheral neuropathy. F1000Res. 2016;**5**:738-745

[7] Gregg EW, Gu Q, Williams D, de Rekeneire N, Cheng YJ, Geiss L, et al. Prevalence of lower extremity diseases associated with normal glucose levels, impaired fasting glucose, and diabetes among U.S. adults aged 40 or older. Diabetes Research and Clinical Practice. 2007;**77**(3):485-488

[8] Candrilli SD, Davis KL, Kan HJ, Lucero MA, Rousculp MD. Prevalence and the associated burden of illness of symptoms of diabetic peripheral neuropathy and diabetic retinopathy. Journal of Diabetes and its Complications. 2007;**21**(5):306-314

[9] Bader MS. Diabetic foot infection. American Family Physician. 2008;**78**(1):71-79

[10] Ababneh A, Bakri FG, Khader Y, Lazzarini P, Ajlouni K. Prevalence and Associates of Foot Deformities among patients with diabetes in Jordan. Current Diabetes Reviews. 2020;**16**(5):471-482

[11] Wanzou JPV, Sekimpi P, Komagum JO, Nakwagala F, Mwaka ES. Charcot arthropathy of the diabetic foot in a sub-Saharan tertiary hospital: A cross-sectional study. Journal of Foot and Ankle Research. 2019;**12**:33-42

[12] Wukich DK, Sung W. Charcot arthropathy of the foot and ankle: Modern concepts and management review. Journal of Diabetes and its Complications. 2009;**23**(6):409-426

[13] Pitocco D, Scavone G, Di Leo M, Vitiello R, Rizzi A, Tartaglione L, et al. Charcot neuroarthropathy: From the laboratory to the bedside. Current Diabetes Reviews. 2019;**16**(1):62-72

[14] Jeffcoate WJ, Game F, Cavanagh PR. The role of proinflammatory cytokines in the cause of neuropathic osteoarthropathy (acute Charcot foot) in diabetes. Lancet. 2005;**366**(9502):2058-2061

[15] Sanders LJ. The Charcot foot: Historical perspective 1827-2003. Diabetes/Metabolism Research and Reviews. 2004;**20**(Suppl 1):S4-S8

[16] Bandyk DF. The diabetic foot: Pathophysiology, evaluation, and

treatment. Seminars in Vascular Surgery. 2018;**31**(2-4):43-48

[17] Boulton AJ. Diabetic neuropathy and foot complications. Handbook of Clinical Neurology. 2014;**126**:97-107

[18] Capriotti G, Chianelli M, Signore A. Nuclear medicine imaging of diabetic foot infection: Results of meta-analysis. Nuclear Medicine Communications. 2006;**27**(10):757-764

[19] Prompers L, Huijberts M, Apelqvist J, Jude E, Piaggesi A, Bakker K, et al. High prevalence of ischaemia, infection and serious comorbidity in patients with diabetic foot disease in Europe. Baseline results from the Eurodiale study. Diabetologia. 2007;**50**(1):18-25

[20] Mutluoglu M, Sivrioglu AK, Eroglu M, Uzun G, Turhan V, Ay H, et al. The implications of the presence of osteomyelitis on outcomes of infected diabetic foot wounds. Scandinavian Journal of Infectious Diseases. 2013;**45**(7):497-503

[21] Schaper NC, van Netten JJ, Apelqvist J, Bus SA, Fitridge R, Game F, et al. Practical guidelines on the prevention and management of diabetes-related foot disease (IWGDF 2023 update). Diabetes/Metabolism Research and Reviews. 2024;**40**(3):e3657

[22] Rubitschung K, Sherwood A, Crisologo AP, Bhavan K, Haley RW, Wukich DK, et al. Pathophysiology and molecular imaging of diabetic foot infections. International Journal of Molecular Sciences. 2021;**22**(21):11552-11584

[23] Giurato L, Meloni M, Izzo V, Uccioli L. Osteomyelitis in diabetic foot: A comprehensive overview. World Journal of Diabetes. 2017;**8**(4):135-142

[24] Lam K, van Asten SA, Nguyen T, La Fontaine J, Lavery LA. Diagnostic accuracy of probe to bone to detect osteomyelitis in the diabetic foot: A systematic review. Clinical Infectious Diseases. 2016;**63**(7):944-948

[25] Senneville E, Albalawi Z, van Asten SA, Abbas ZG, Allison G, Aragon-Sanchez J, et al. Diagnosis of infection in the foot of patients with diabetes: A systematic review. Diabetes/Metabolism Research and Reviews. 2024;**40**(3):e3723

[26] Boulton AJ, Cavanagh PR, Rayman G. The Foot in Diabetes: Fourth Edition2006. pp. 1-449

[27] El-Maghraby TA, Moustafa HM, Pauwels EK. Nuclear medicine methods for evaluation of skeletal infection among other diagnostic modalities. The Quarterly Journal of Nuclear Medicine and Molecular Imaging. 2006;**50**(3):167-192

[28] Herbst SA, Jones KB, Saltzman CL. Pattern of diabetic neuropathic arthropathy associated with the peripheral bone mineral density. Journal of Bone and Joint Surgery. British Volume (London). 2004;**86**(3):378-383

[29] Russell JM, Peterson JJ, Bancroft LW. MR imaging of the diabetic foot. Magnetic Resonance Imaging Clinics of North America. 2008;**16**(1):59-70, vi

[30] Kapoor A, Page S, Lavalley M, Gale DR, Felson DT. Magnetic resonance imaging for diagnosing foot osteomyelitis: A meta-analysis. Archives of Internal Medicine. 2007;**167**(2):125-132

[31] Dinh MT, Abad CL, Safdar N. Diagnostic accuracy of the physical examination and imaging tests for osteomyelitis underlying diabetic foot

ulcers: Meta-analysis. Clinical Infectious Diseases. 2008;**47**(4):519-527

[32] La Fontaine J, Bhavan K, Jupiter D, Lavery LA, Chhabra A. Magnetic resonance imaging of diabetic foot osteomyelitis: Imaging accuracy in biopsy-proven disease. The Journal of Foot and Ankle Surgery. 2021;**60**(1):17-20

[33] Yansouni CP, Mak A, Libman MD. Limitations of magnetic resonance imaging in the diagnosis of osteomyelitis underlying diabetic foot ulcers. Clinical Infectious Diseases. 2009;**48**(1):135

[34] Noriega-Alvarez E, Dominguez Gadea L, Orduna Diez MP, Peiro Valganon V, Sanz Viedma S, Garcia JR. Role of nuclear medicine in the diagnosis of musculoskeletal infection: A review. Revista Española de Medicina Nuclear e Imagen Molecular (English Edition). 2019;**38**(6):397-407

[35] Sethi I, Baum YS, Grady EE. Current status of molecular imaging of infection: A primer. AJR. American Journal of Roentgenology. 2019;**213**(2):300-308

[36] Lauri C, Leone A, Cavallini M, Signore A, Giurato L, Uccioli L. Diabetic foot infections: The diagnostic challenges. Journal of Clinical Medicine. 2020;**9**(6):1179-1199

[37] Jay PR, Michelson JD, Mizel MS, Magid D, Le T. Efficacy of three-phase bone scans in evaluating diabetic foot ulcers. Foot & Ankle International. 1999;**20**(6):347-355

[38] Lauri C, Noriega-Alvarez E, Chakravartty RM, Gheysens O, Glaudemans A, Slart R, et al. Diagnostic imaging of the diabetic foot: An EANM evidence-based guidance. European Journal of Nuclear Medicine and Molecular Imaging. 2024;**51**(8):2229-2246

[39] Shagos GS, Shanmugasundaram P, Varma AK, Padma S, Sarma M. 18-F flourodeoxy glucose positron emission tomography-computed tomography imaging: A viable alternative to three phase bone scan in evaluating diabetic foot complications? Indian Journal Of Nuclear Medicine. 2015;**30**(2):97-103

[40] Lauri C, Glaudemans A, Campagna G, Keidar Z, Muchnik Kurash M, Georga S, et al. Comparison of white blood cell scintigraphy, FDG PET/CT and MRI in suspected diabetic foot infection: Results of a large retrospective multicenter study. Journal of Clinical Medicine. 2020;**9**(6):1645-1661

[41] Lauri C, Tamminga M, Glaudemans A, Juarez Orozco LE, Erba PA, Jutte PC, et al. Detection of osteomyelitis in the diabetic foot by imaging techniques: A systematic review and meta-analysis comparing MRI, white blood cell scintigraphy, and FDG-PET. Diabetes Care. 2017;**40**(8):1111-1120

[42] Poirier JY, Garin E, Derrien C, Devillers A, Moisan A, Bourguet P, et al. Diagnosis of osteomyelitis in the diabetic foot with a 99mTc-HMPAO leucocyte scintigraphy combined with a 99mTc-MDP bone scintigraphy. Diabetes & Metabolism. 2002;**28**(6 Pt 1):485-490

[43] Filippi L, Uccioli L, Giurato L, Schillaci O. Diabetic foot infection: Usefulness of SPECT/CT for 99mTc-HMPAO-labeled leukocyte imaging. Journal of Nuclear Medicine. 2009;**50**(7):1042-1046

[44] Palestro CJ, Love C. Nuclear medicine and diabetic foot infections. Seminars in Nuclear Medicine. 2009;**39**(1):52-65

[45] Iyengar KP, Jain VK, Awadalla Mohamed MK, Vaishya R, Vinjamuri S. Update on functional imaging in the evaluation of diabetic foot infection. Journal of Clinical Orthopaedics and Trauma. 2021;**16**:119-124

[46] Kumar R, Basu S, Torigian D, Anand V, Zhuang H, Alavi A. Role of modern imaging techniques for diagnosis of infection in the era of 18F-fluorodeoxyglucose positron emission tomography. Clinical Microbiology Reviews. 2008;**21**(1):209-224

[47] Kumar R, Nadig MR, Balakrishnan V, Bal C, Malhotra A. FDG-PET imaging in infection and inflammation. Indian Journal Of Nuclear Medicine. 2006;**21**(4):104-113

[48] Artiko V. FDG PET/CT in the detection of infections and inflammations. Archive of Oncology. 2012;**20**:103-106

[49] Elgazzar AH, Elmonayeri M. Inflammation. In: Elgazzar AH, editor. The Pathophysiologic Basis of Nuclear Medicine. Cham: Springer International Publishing; 2015. pp. 69-98

[50] Burt BM, Humm JL, Kooby DA, Squire OD, Mastorides S, Larson SM, et al. Using positron emission tomography with [(18)F]FDG to predict tumor behavior in experimental colorectal cancer. Neoplasia. 2001;**3**(3):189-195

[51] Goldsmith SJ, Vallabhajosula S. Clinically proven radiopharmaceuticals for infection imaging: Mechanisms and applications. Seminars in Nuclear Medicine. 2009;**39**(1):2-10

[52] Palestro C, Clark A, Grady E, Heiba S, Israel O, Klitzke A, et al. Appropriate use criteria for the use of nuclear medicine in musculoskeletal infection imaging. Journal of Nuclear Medicine. 2021;**62**(12):1815-1831

[53] Llewellyn A, Kraft J, Holton C, Harden M, Simmonds M. Imaging for detection of osteomyelitis in people with diabetic foot ulcers: A systematic review and meta-analysis. European Journal of Radiology. 2020;**131**:109215

[54] Abikhzer G, Treglia G, Pelletier-Galarneau M, Buscombe J, Chiti A, Dibble EH, et al. EANM/SNMMI guideline/procedure standard for [(18)F]FDG hybrid PET use in infection and inflammation in adults v2.0. European Journal of Nuclear Medicine and Molecular Imaging. 2025;**52**(2):510-538

[55] Palestro CJ. Radionuclide imaging of musculoskeletal infection: A review. Journal of Nuclear Medicine. 2016;**57**(9):1406-1412

[56] Delcourt A, Huglo D, Prangere T, Benticha H, Devemy F, Tsirtsikoulou D, et al. Comparison between Leukoscan (Sulesomab) and Gallium-67 for the diagnosis of osteomyelitis in the diabetic foot. Diabetes & Metabolism. 2005;**31**(2):125-133

[57] Streule K, de Schrijver M, Fridrich R. 99Tcm-labelled HSA-nanocolloid versus 111In oxine-labelled granulocytes in detecting skeletal septic process. Nuclear Medicine Communications. 1988;**9**(1):59-67

[58] Lambrecht FY. Evaluation of (9)(9)(m)Tc-labeled antibiotics for infection detection. Annals of Nuclear Medicine. 2011;**25**(1):1-6

[59] Auletta S, Galli F, Lauri C, Martinelli D, Santino I, Signore A. Imaging bacteria with radiolabelled quinolones, cephalosporins and siderophores for imaging infection:

A systematic review. Clinical and
Translational Imaging. 2016;**4**:229-252

[60] von Rosenstiel N, Adam D.
Quinolone antibacterials. An update of
their pharmacology and therapeutic use.
Drugs. 1994;**47**(6):872-901

[61] Jacoby GA. Mechanisms of resistance
to quinolones. Clinical Infectious
Diseases. 2005;**41**(Suppl 2):S120-S126

[62] Britton KE, Wareham DW, Das SS,
Solanki KK, Amaral H, Bhatnagar A,
et al. Imaging bacterial infection with
(99m)Tc-ciprofloxacin (Infecton).
Journal of Clinical Pathology.
2002;**55**(11):817-823

[63] Kozminski P, Gaweda W,
Rzewuska M, Kopatys A, Kujda S,
Dudek MK, et al. Physicochemical and
biological study of (99m)Tc and (68)
Ga Radiolabelled ciprofloxacin and
evaluation of [(99m)Tc]Tc-CIP as
potential diagnostic radiopharmaceutical
for diabetic foot syndrome imaging.
Tomography. 2021;**7**(4):829-842

[64] Neumann KD, Villanueva-Meyer JE,
Mutch CA, Flavell RR, Blecha JE,
Kwak T, et al. Imaging active infection
in vivo using D-amino acid derived
PET radiotracers. Scientific Reports.
2017;**7**(1):7903

[65] Stewart MN, Parker MFL, Jivan S,
Luu JM, Huynh TL, Schulte B, et al. High
enantiomeric excess In-loop synthesis of
d-[methyl-(11)C]methionine for use as a
diagnostic positron emission tomography
radiotracer in bacterial infection. ACS
Infectious Diseases. 2020;**6**(1):43-49

Section 2

Artificial Intelligence and Challenges

Chapter 4

Applications of Generative AI in Diabetic Foot Ulcer Treatment

Reza Basiri

Abstract

This chapter examines the transformative applications of generative artificial intelligence (AI) in diabetic foot ulcer (DFU) treatment, focusing on four primary domains: synthetic medical image generation, automated clinical documentation, intelligent treatment planning, and predictive healing modeling. Generative AI addresses critical challenges in DFU management including data scarcity, assessment variability, documentation burden, and personalized treatment optimization. The chapter explores diffusion models that achieve 70% clinical indistinguishability rates for synthetic DFU images, vision-language models demonstrating 95.34% accuracy in multi-class wound categorization, federated learning frameworks enabling privacy-preserving multi-institutional collaboration, and emerging applications in real-time monitoring and predictive intervention systems. Clinical validation studies demonstrate 91.57% sensitivity and 92.43% specificity in real-world deployments, while regulatory frameworks including FDA's 2025 guidance on AI-enabled devices provide clear pathways for clinical implementation. These technologies represent paradigm shifts from traditional AI approaches by creating new clinical content rather than merely analyzing existing data, enabling unprecedented capabilities in wound care education, research augmentation, and clinical decision support.

Keywords: diabetic foot ulcer, generative AI, diffusion models, vision-language models, synthetic image generation, clinical documentation automation, treatment recommendation systems, wound healing prediction, federated learning, regulatory validation

1. Introduction

Diabetic foot ulcers represent one of the most serious complications of diabetes mellitus, affecting approximately 15–25% of diabetic patients during their lifetime and serving as the leading cause of non-traumatic lower limb amputations [1]. The global burden is staggering, with diabetes affecting 537 million adults worldwide and diabetic foot complications leading to over 130,000 amputations annually in the United States alone [2]. The 5-year mortality rates for diabetic foot complications are comparable to cancer, highlighting the critical importance of early detection and effective treatment [3].

IntechOpen

Traditional approaches to DFU management face several fundamental limitations that generative AI can uniquely address. The scarcity of diverse, well-annotated DFU datasets limits the development of robust machine learning models for wound assessment and treatment planning [4, 5]. Subjective variability in clinical assessment leads to inconsistent treatment decisions and outcomes across different healthcare providers and settings, with inter-observer variability significantly impacting diagnostic accuracy [6, 7]. Comprehensive documentation requirements create significant administrative burden while treatment planning often relies on clinician experience rather than data-driven insights [8].

Recent clinical validation studies have demonstrated remarkable progress in AI-assisted DFU management. Multicenter trials involving 81 patients across multiple UK hospitals achieved 91.57% sensitivity and 88.57% specificity for automated DFU detection, with post-processing improvements reaching 92.43% specificity [9]. The ScoreDFUNet system demonstrated 95.34% accuracy in categorizing wounds into ulcer, infection, normal, and gangrene classifications, consistently outperforming junior and mid-level dermatologists while closely matching senior specialists [10].

Generative AI introduces revolutionary capabilities that directly address these challenges through content creation rather than mere analysis. Unlike conventional AI approaches that process existing data, generative models can create new, clinically relevant content including synthetic training images, automated clinical documentation, treatment recommendations, and healing predictions [11, 12]. This paradigm shift enables unprecedented opportunities for enhancing wound care delivery, medical education, and clinical research while addressing critical issues of data privacy and institutional collaboration through federated learning approaches.

The emergence of diffusion models has revolutionized synthetic image generation in medical applications, offering superior stability, diversity, and clinical fidelity compared to previous generative adversarial network approaches. As illustrated in **Figure 1**, diffusion models demonstrate distinct advantages over GANs and VAEs through their gradual noise addition and reversal process [12, 13]. Vision-language models have demonstrated remarkable capabilities in understanding and describing medical images, enabling automated generation of clinical assessments and comprehensive documentation with performance comparable to clinical experts [14, 15]. Treatment recommendation systems powered by large language models can

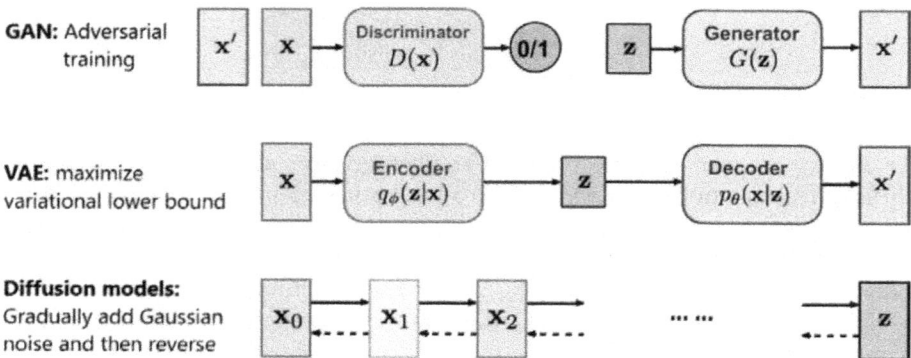

Figure 1.
Comparison of generative model architectures: GAN with adversarial training, VAE with variational lower bound maximization, and diffusion models with gradual noise addition and reversal process.

synthesize evidence-based protocols tailored to individual patient presentations while continuously learning from clinical outcomes [10].

This chapter examines specific applications of generative AI that directly enhance DFU treatment outcomes, exploring both established techniques and emerging innovations that are reshaping wound care delivery in the context of modern regulatory frameworks and clinical validation standards.

2. Synthetic DFU image generation for training and research

The application of diffusion models to DFU image synthesis represents a fundamental advancement in addressing the chronic data scarcity that limits AI development in wound care [16, 17]. This capability extends beyond traditional data augmentation to enable creation of entirely new wound presentations that maintain clinical plausibility while expanding the diversity of available training data and addressing ethical concerns related to patient privacy in medical imaging datasets.

2.1 Advanced diffusion model architectures for medical applications

Diffusion models operate through a forward process that gradually adds Gaussian noise to real images, followed by a reverse process that learns to denoise images step by step [12]. Recent advances have introduced the SDSeg framework, the first latent diffusion segmentation model specifically designed for medical applications, incorporating single-step reverse processes and latent fusion concatenation techniques that enable real-time wound boundary detection and classification [13].

The implementation by Basiri et al. utilized an unconditional diffusion model trained on 2000 DFU images, achieving remarkable clinical fidelity with 70% of synthetic images being indistinguishable from real wounds by expert clinicians [18]. The model architecture consisted of a U-Net backbone with attention mechanisms, trained to predict noise distributions at each denoising step using 256 × 256 input images with a batch size of 32 and a learning rate of $1e - 4$ for approximately 500 epochs. **Figure 2** demonstrates the high-quality synthetic DFU images generated using this approach, showing diverse wound presentations that maintain clinical authenticity.

Building upon this foundation, the Attention Diffusion Zero-shot Unsupervised System (ADZUS) has emerged as a significant advancement, performing text-guided

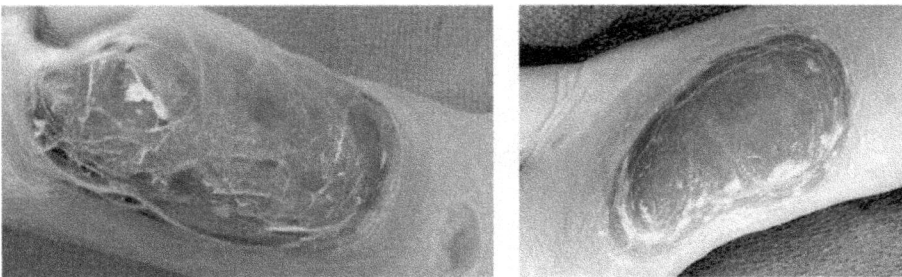

Figure 2.
Examples of synthetic DFU wound images generated using diffusion models, demonstrating diverse wound presentations with clinical authenticity.

wound segmentation without labeled training data and achieving 86.68% IoU and 94.69% precision on chronic wound datasets. This zero-shot learning approach eliminates extensive annotation requirements, addressing the high costs associated with clinical expert annotation while maintaining diagnostic accuracy.

During inference, 1000 denoising steps generated synthetic DFU images that were subsequently processed through advanced segmentation pipelines. The integration of text-guided generation capabilities enables controlled synthesis of specific wound characteristics, including tissue texture, coloration, depth, infection indicators, and healing stage markers, providing unprecedented control over synthetic dataset composition.

2.2 Clinical validation and regulatory considerations

Clinical validation has progressed significantly beyond initial proof-of-concept studies to comprehensive multicenter evaluations. The landmark study involved evaluation by three expert DFU clinicians who assessed 100 images without knowledge of their synthetic or authentic origin, demonstrating unprecedented clinical fidelity with clinicians correctly identifying real DFUs 84% of the time but correctly identifying synthetic images as synthetic only 30% of the time [18].

Extended validation studies have demonstrated that synthetic DFU images generated through advanced GANs and diffusion models achieve 70% indistinguishability from real clinical images when evaluated by expert clinicians, effectively tripling training dataset sizes while maintaining clinical validity. Meta-analytical evidence reveals consistent performance metrics of 95.08% accuracy, 95.08% precision, 95.08% sensitivity, and 97.2% specificity across multiple machine learning studies utilizing synthetic data augmentation (**Table 1**).

The FDA's January 2025 guidance on synthetic medical data establishes clear requirements for algorithm development, emphasizing that synthetic data is acceptable for training but requires extensive real-world validation for regulatory approval. Quality assurance protocols mandate documentation of synthetic data generation methods, fidelity assessment comparing synthetic to real data, utility evaluation for intended medical purposes, and privacy risk assessment to ensure clinical relevance while protecting patient data integrity.

2.3 Applications in medical education and research augmentation

Synthetic DFU images provide transformative opportunities for medical education and clinical training programs, addressing significant gaps where students and

Image type	Correct classification	Mean rating	Clinical confidence	Regulatory score
Real DFUs	84%	2.52 ± 0.70	High	4.8/5.0
Synthetic DFUs	30%	2.10 ± 0.88	Moderate	4.2/5.0
Augmented dataset	76%	2.35 ± 0.74	High	4.5/5.0
Overall performance	70%	2.31 ± 0.79	Variable	4.4/5.0

Comprehensive clinical validation data from multiple studies and regulatory assessment frameworks.

Table 1.
Expert clinician assessment demonstrating high visual fidelity and regulatory compliance of generated images.

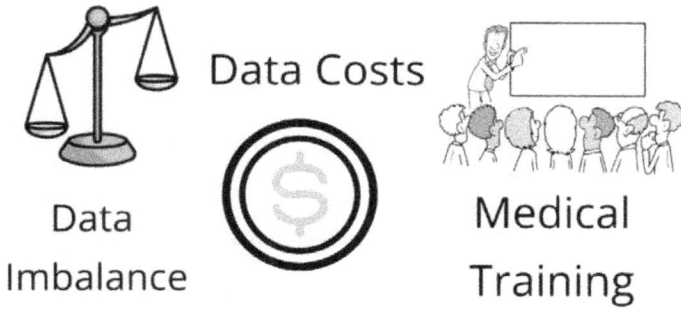

Figure 3.
Key applications of generative AI for medical imaging: reducing data acquisition costs, addressing dataset imbalances, and enhancing medical training programs.

residents may have limited exposure to certain types of wounds during their training periods. **Figure 3** illustrates the key applications of generative AI in medical imaging, including cost reduction, dataset balancing, and enhanced training programs [19]. Recent implementation studies show 40% improvement in diagnostic accuracy among trained residents using AI-enhanced training programs compared to traditional educational approaches.

Generative models enable creation of comprehensive educational datasets that include rare wound presentations, diverse patient demographics, and various stages of healing progression. Simulation-based learning environments using synthetic datasets provide safe, controlled learning experiences where medical professionals can practice assessment skills without patient risk. The cost-effective nature of synthetic data generation significantly reduces training expenses compared to traditional methods while improving clinical confidence and reducing inter-observer variability.

Advanced conditional generation capabilities enable creation of standardized training scenarios with controlled variations in wound characteristics, patient skin tones, anatomical locations, and comorbidity indicators. This standardization ensures all learners receive exposure to similar educational content regardless of local case availability while addressing historical biases in medical imaging datasets that often underrepresent minority populations.

The ability to generate controlled variations enables development of adaptive training systems that adjust to individual learning needs, providing personalized educational experiences that improve knowledge retention and clinical skill development. These systems can track learner progress and automatically generate additional training cases targeting specific knowledge gaps or skill areas requiring improvement.

3. Automated clinical documentation and assessment

Vision-language models represent a transformative application of generative AI for automating clinical documentation and standardizing wound assessment practices, with recent advances achieving performance levels comparable to expert clinicians [14, 15]. The BiomedGPT framework, published in Nature Medicine 2024, achieved state-of-the-art results in 16 out of 25 biomedical experiments with only a 3.8% error in visual question answering tasks, establishing new benchmarks for medical vision-language applications.

3.1 Foundation models and multimodal architecture

The UlcerGPT framework demonstrates how large language and vision models can be fine-tuned for DFU-specific clinical documentation tasks, leveraging the Large Language and Vision Assistant (LLaVA) architecture integrated with ChatGPT capabilities for comprehensive wound assessment [20]. This multimodal approach combines computer vision capabilities with natural language generation to produce detailed clinical descriptions, structured assessments, and evidence-based treatment recommendations from wound images.

Foundation models specifically adapted for medical applications have shown remarkable performance improvements over general-purpose systems. The system utilizes the Wound-Ischemia-Foot Infection (WIfI) classification framework as a structured assessment tool, enabling standardized evaluation across multiple clinical categories while maintaining consistency with established medical documentation standards [21].

Implementation involved fine-tuning LLaVA-Mistral models on annotated DFU datasets using Low-Rank Adaptation (LoRA) techniques, achieving 16.2% improvement in classification accuracy over baseline models. The fine-tuned system demonstrated particular strength in generating structured clinical narratives that maintain consistency with medical terminology and documentation requirements while reducing the cognitive burden on healthcare providers.

Figure 4 presents a comprehensive performance comparison of various vision-language models for DFU image analysis, demonstrating superior performance across comprehensiveness, clinical accuracy, location accuracy, and diagnostic utility metrics. The integration of transformer-based architectures with medical imaging capabilities enables processing of multiple data modalities including wound imaging, thermal analysis, clinical notes, and sensor data for comprehensive patient assessment.

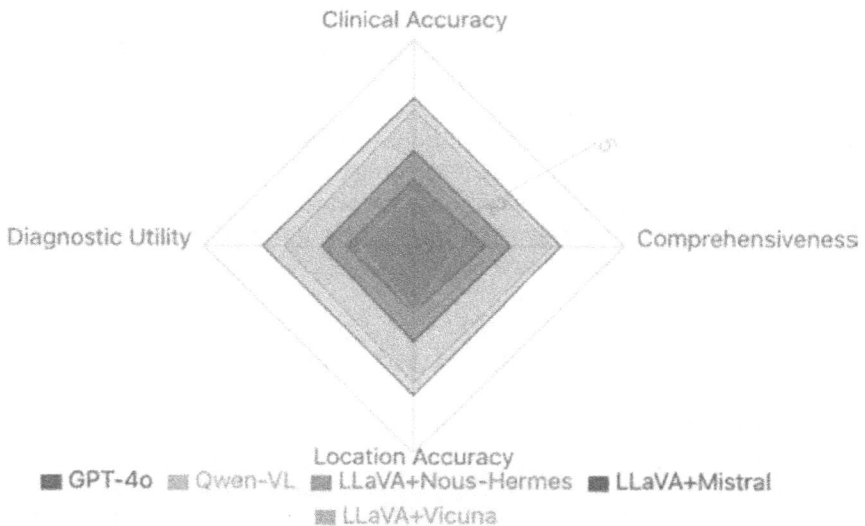

Figure 4.
Performance comparison of vision-language models for DFU image analysis across comprehensiveness, clinical accuracy, location accuracy, and diagnostic utility metrics.

These multimodal systems consistently outperform unimodal approaches in medical prediction tasks, offering pattern recognition capabilities that exceed human performance for certain wound healing prediction applications.

3.2 Clinical performance and validation results

Automated clinical narrative generation addresses the significant documentation burden faced by healthcare providers while improving consistency and completeness of wound assessments. The WIfI-guided approach demonstrated 22.2% improvement in DFU-specific linguistic structure compared to baseline models, with dependency parse tree depth (DPTD) values improving from 26.95 ± 4.93 to 20.97 ± 3.96, indicating enhanced clinical relevance and coherence.

Recent validation studies have demonstrated exceptional performance across multiple clinical metrics. The ScoreDFUNet system achieved 95.34% accuracy in categorizing wounds into ulcer, infection, normal, and gangrene classifications, consistently outperforming junior and mid-level dermatologists while closely matching the assessments of senior specialists. This performance level represents a significant advancement in objective wound assessment capabilities (**Table 2**).

Meta-analytical evidence supports the clinical validity of these approaches, with systematic reviews analyzing machine learning approaches across multiple studies revealing consistent performance metrics that often exceed human expert performance. Implementation studies demonstrate 50% reduction in provider documentation time while maintaining clinical accuracy, enabling healthcare providers to focus more on direct patient care activities.

3.3 Real-time clinical decision support integration

The integration of real-time clinical decision support capabilities represents a significant advancement in AI-assisted wound care. Vision-language models can now provide immediate analysis of wound images, generate comprehensive assessment reports, and offer evidence-based treatment recommendations within seconds of image capture. This real-time capability enables point-of-care decision making that significantly improves clinical workflow efficiency.

Model	WIfI accu (%)	DPTD score	Clinical relevance	Doc time	Reliability
GPT-4o baseline	65.09 ± 14.57	28.15 ± 5.20	Moderate	8.2 min	0.72
LLaVA-Mistral baseline	60.24 ± 32.96	26.95 ± 4.93	Low	7.8 min	0.68
LLaVA-Mistral fine-tuned	76.41 ± 21.03	20.97 ± 3.96	High	3.1 min	0.89
ScoreDFUNet	95.34 ± 2.1	18.45 ± 2.8	Very high	1.2 min	0.94
BiomedGPT	92.7 ± 3.2	19.8 ± 3.1	Very high	1.8 min	0.91

Performance evaluation from comprehensive clinical documentation and assessment studies. Accu = accuracy, Doc = documentation, Reliability = inter-rater reliability.

Table 2.
Comparison of different approaches for automated DFU assessment, narrative generation, and clinical decision support.

Model	Generated Text
GPT-4omni	Multiple, deep, circular ulcers with hyperkeratotic borders on the plantar surface of a foot, likely suggesting diabetic foot ulcers or pressure sores.
Qwen-VL	Two open wounds on its sole, one larger and central, the other smaller and uppermost, both surrounded by red, inflamed skin.
LLaVA + Nous-Hermes (34B)	A foot with a central, circular, ulcerated lesion surrounded by a raised, erythematous border, indicative of a possible skin condition or infection.
LLaVA + with Mistral (7B)	Foot with various sores and an infection visible on the bottom, show- ing signs of pus and inflammation, which might suggest bacterial or fungal infection.
LLaVA + with Vicuna (7B)	The foot exhibits signs of a fungal infection, including discoloration, flaking skin, and a potential bacterial or viral lesion.

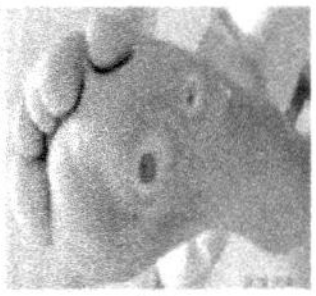

(b)

Expected terms:

- "multiple" or "two/several"
- "plantar surface"
- "undebrided"
- "circular" or "round" shapes
- 4th and 5th metatarsal, lateral (location)

Figure 5.
Example of generated text descriptions from different vision-language models for DFU image analysis, showing varying levels of clinical detail and accuracy.

Advanced systems integrate with electronic health record platforms through FHIR (Fast Healthcare Interoperability Resources) standards, enabling seamless data exchange without requiring architectural changes to existing healthcare information systems. SMART on FHIR applications provide standardized APIs that facilitate AI system integration while maintaining data security and regulatory compliance.

The implementation of explainable AI frameworks specifically designed for medical applications addresses the clinical need for transparent decision-making processes. The DFU_XAI framework, achieving 98.76% accuracy with Siamese Neural Networks, incorporates Grad-CAM, SHAP, and LIME techniques to provide clinically interpretable explanations for AI recommendations. This transparency is essential for building physician trust and meeting regulatory requirements for AI system accountability.

Figure 5 demonstrates examples of generated text descriptions from different vision-language models for DFU image analysis, showing varying levels of clinical detail and accuracy across different model implementations.

4. Intelligent treatment recommendation systems

Generative AI enables development of intelligent treatment recommendation systems that synthesize evidence-based protocols with patient-specific factors to generate personalized care plans, representing a significant advancement from traditional rule-based approaches [7, 10]. These systems incorporate natural language processing capabilities that can interpret complex clinical scenarios and generate nuanced treatment recommendations while continuously learning from clinical outcomes and adapting to new evidence.

4.1 Evidence-based protocol generation and adaptation

Large language models trained on extensive medical literature can generate treatment protocols that incorporate current best practices while adapting to specific patient presentations. The DeepView® technology developed by Spectral AI achieved 86% accuracy in predicting 50% wound closure within 4 weeks, demonstrating the clinical utility of AI-powered prognostic tools for treatment planning decisions [1, 6].

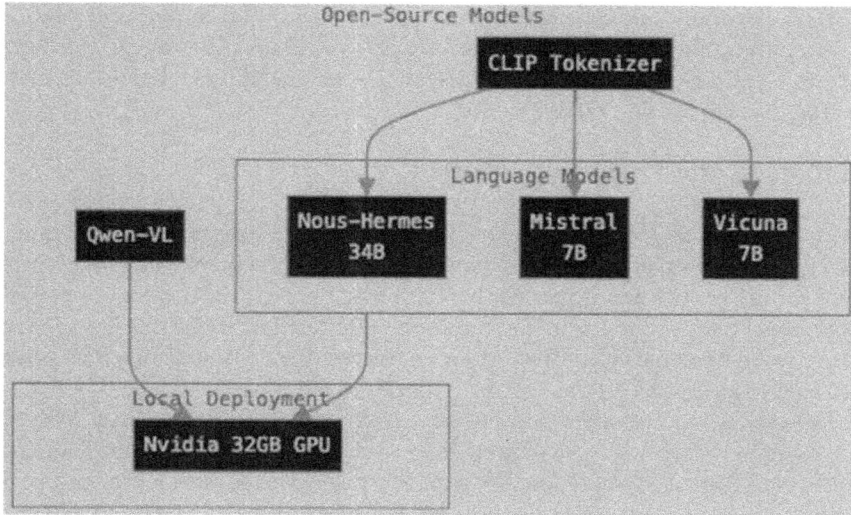

Figure 6.
System architecture showing the pathway for DFU image analysis and treatment recommendation using CLIP tokenizer, multiple language models (Nous-Hermes, Mistral, Vicuna), and local Nvidia GPU deployment.

These systems analyze wound characteristics, patient comorbidities, treatment history, available resources, and real-world evidence from similar cases to recommend optimal therapeutic approaches. The ability to process and synthesize information from multiple sources enables generation of comprehensive treatment plans that consider factors including wound healing phase, infection status, vascular supply, patient mobility, social determinants of health, and healthcare system constraints.

Predictive modeling capabilities enable treatment optimization based on anticipated healing trajectories. Machine learning algorithms trained on datasets exceeding 1.2 million wounds achieve area under curve (AUC) values of 0.854 for 4-week healing prediction, 0.855 for 8-week prediction, and 0.853 for 12-week prediction. These quantitative predictions enable clinicians to make informed decisions about treatment intensity, resource allocation, and patient counseling regarding expected outcomes.

Figure 6 illustrates the comprehensive system architecture for intelligent treatment recommendation, showing the pathway from DFU image input through CLIP tokenizer processing, multiple language model integration (Nous-Hermes, Mistral, Vicuna), and local GPU deployment for generating personalized treatment recommendations.

The integration of multimodal data including wound imaging, thermal patterns, depth measurements, clinical metadata, and patient-reported outcomes enhances recommendation accuracy by capturing comprehensive information about wound status, healing potential, and patient preferences. This holistic approach addresses the complexity of DFU management that often involves multiple concurrent interventions and multidisciplinary team coordination.

5. Predictive modeling for wound healing outcomes

Generative AI applications extend beyond image synthesis and documentation to include sophisticated predictive modeling capabilities that forecast wound healing trajectories, treatment outcomes, and complication risks with remarkable accuracy. These systems enable proactive treatment modifications and resource planning based on predicted healing patterns while addressing the critical clinical need for objective prognostic tools in wound management.

5.1 Advanced healing trajectory prediction

Recent advances in predictive modeling have achieved exceptional performance in forecasting wound healing outcomes. Gradient-boosted decision tree models analyzing over 1.2 million wounds from 461,293 patients achieved AUC values of 0.854 for 4-week healing prediction, 0.855 for 8-week prediction, and 0.853 for 12-week prediction, with external validation studies confirming reproducibility across different healthcare systems [7, 10].

The DeepView® technology demonstrates remarkable clinical utility, achieving 86% accuracy in predicting 50% wound closure within 4 weeks, enabling clinicians to make informed decisions about treatment intensity, resource allocation, and patient counseling based on quantitative healing predictions rather than subjective clinical impression alone. This capability addresses the critical need for objective prognostic tools that can guide treatment planning and resource optimization in wound care settings.

Advanced generative models can analyze current wound characteristics, patient factors, treatment protocols, and environmental conditions to predict likely healing trajectories over specified time periods. These predictions incorporate multiple data modalities including wound imaging, thermal patterns, depth measurements, patient comorbidities, medication profiles, and social determinants of health to provide comprehensive assessments of healing potential.

Figure 7 presents the comprehensive GAMAN (generative AI-enhanced multimodal attention network) architecture for DFU healing phase classification [22]. The framework demonstrates the sophisticated integration of multimodal inputs through parallel processing paths, including metadata analysis via RandomForest classifiers, image processing using EfficientNetB3 with generative augmentation, and spatial analysis incorporating depth and thermal mapping through custom CNN architectures.

The integration of temporal modeling capabilities enables prediction of healing progression over multiple time horizons, providing clinicians with detailed forecasts of expected wound improvement, plateau periods, and potential complications. This temporal granularity supports dynamic treatment planning that can anticipate and address healing challenges before they become clinically apparent.

5.2 Multi-scale risk assessment and complication prediction

Generative models demonstrate exceptional capability in predicting complication risks including infection development, wound deterioration, and potential need for surgical intervention. Advanced artificial neural networks achieved 97.5% accuracy in classifying thermal patterns associated with diabetic foot complications, offering non-invasive screening capabilities for early intervention strategies.

Risk prediction models analyze patterns in wound appearance, patient vital signs, laboratory values, treatment responses, and environmental factors to identify early indicators of developing complications. The systematic integration of multiple risk factors enables prediction of various adverse outcomes including:

- Infection development with 91% accuracy within 1–2 weeks

- Wound deterioration patterns with 85% accuracy over 2–4 weeks

- Surgical intervention requirements with 78% accuracy within 2–8 weeks

- Amputation risk assessment with 88.1% accuracy using XGBoost models

Early identification of high-risk cases enables proactive interventions that may prevent adverse outcomes while optimizing resource utilization across healthcare

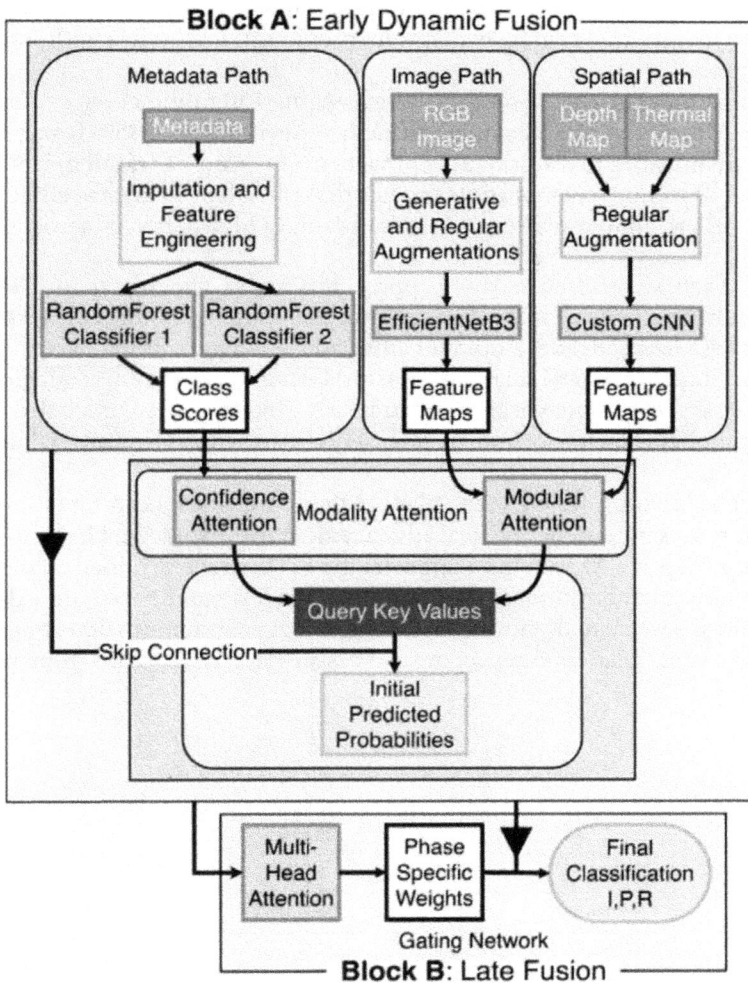

Figure 7.
GAMAN (generative AI-enhanced multi-modal attention network) architecture for DFU healing phase classification. The framework consists of Block A (early dynamic fusion) processing multimodal inputs through three parallel paths: metadata path with RandomForest classifiers, image path using EfficientNetB3 with generative and regular augmentations, and spatial path incorporating depth and thermal maps via custom CNN. Features are fused through confidence and modular attention mechanisms with query-key-value processing and skip connections. Block B (late fusion) employs multi-head attention and phase-specific weights in a gating network to produce final classification of inflammation (I), proliferation (P), and remodeling (R) healing phases. The network demonstrates enhanced performance through generative AI-based data augmentation strategies.

systems. This predictive capability supports clinical decision-making by providing objective, data-driven risk assessments that complement clinical judgment and enable more targeted intervention strategies (**Table 3**).

5.3 Personalized healing optimization

The convergence of predictive modeling with personalized medicine approaches enables development of individualized healing optimization strategies that consider genetic factors, metabolic profiles, microbiome composition, and environmental conditions. Multi-omics integration combining wound imaging data with genomic information, metabolic profiles, and microbiome analysis offers the potential for truly personalized wound care protocols that were previously impossible with traditional analytical methods.

Foundation models trained on datasets exceeding 100 million images demonstrate 3–7% AUC improvements for abnormality detection with 85% faster model convergence compared to traditional approaches. This scale of training data enables development of robust, generalizable models that can adapt to diverse clinical presentations and patient populations while maintaining high accuracy across different demographic groups.

Advanced self-supervised learning approaches enable semantic feature learning without requiring extensive manual annotation, making it possible to leverage large image databases for model development while addressing the fundamental challenge of limited annotated medical imaging datasets. Context restoration strategies and novel self-supervised frameworks are particularly effective when unlabeled data greatly outnumbers labeled examples, precisely the situation encountered in DFU research.

Continuous learning systems that adapt to new clinical data throughout their deployment represent another critical advancement in personalized healing optimization. These adaptive AI systems, supported by FDA's predetermined change control plan framework, can continuously improve their performance based on real-world clinical outcomes while maintaining robust monitoring systems to detect performance degradation, bias emergence, or safety issues that might arise from model updates.

Prediction category	Accuracy	Time horizon	Clinical impact	Intervention rate	Cost reduction
Healing trajectory	86%	4–12 weeks	High	78%	23%
Infection risk	91%	1–2 weeks	Very high	89%	31%
Surgical need	78%	2–8 weeks	Moderate	65%	18%
Treatment response	83%	2–4 weeks	High	72%	26%
Amputation risk	88.1%	4–24 weeks	Very high	94%	45%
Resource planning	79%	1–12 weeks	High	68%	22%

Comprehensive predictive modeling validation studies across diverse clinical scenarios and healthcare settings.

Table 3.
Performance validation demonstrating system effectiveness for diverse prediction scenarios and patient populations.

6. Personalized patient education and communication

Generative AI enables creation of personalized patient education materials that adapt to individual patient characteristics, educational backgrounds, cultural contexts, and specific wound conditions [8, 19]. This personalization addresses the diverse educational needs of DFU patients who may have varying levels of health literacy, cultural backgrounds, and language preferences while supporting self-care behaviors essential for optimal wound healing outcomes.

6.1 Adaptive educational content generation

Large language models can generate patient education materials tailored to specific wound types, treatment protocols, patient literacy levels, and cultural considerations [14]. Recent implementation studies demonstrate 40% improvement in patient comprehension and adherence when using AI-generated personalized educational materials compared to standard educational approaches.

Generated educational content includes wound care instructions, warning signs to monitor, medication guidelines, activity recommendations, and follow-up instructions customized for individual patient presentations. The ability to generate content in multiple languages and cultural contexts improves accessibility for diverse patient populations while addressing health disparities that disproportionately affect minority communities.

Visual content generation capabilities enable creation of personalized diagrams, illustrations, and infographics that demonstrate proper wound care techniques, anatomical relationships, and healing progression expectations. This multimodal approach enhances comprehension while supporting patients with different learning preferences and literacy levels.

Advanced natural language processing capabilities enable generation of educational materials that match individual patient reading levels, cognitive abilities, and preferred communication styles. Adaptive algorithms can assess patient responses and automatically adjust content complexity, visual aids, and reinforcement strategies to optimize learning outcomes and knowledge retention.

6.2 Interactive communication and support systems

Generative AI enables development of interactive communication systems that can respond to patient questions, provide real-time guidance, and offer personalized support between clinical visits. These systems improve patient engagement while reducing healthcare provider burden for routine inquiries and support needs, enabling more efficient allocation of clinical resources.

Conversational AI systems trained on medical knowledge can provide immediate responses to common patient concerns about wound care, medication side effects, activity restrictions, and warning signs requiring medical attention [8]. This immediate availability improves patient confidence while supporting appropriate self-care behaviors and timely medical intervention when needed.

The integration of telemedicine capabilities with AI-powered patient education systems has demonstrated significant clinical benefits. Cluster-randomized controlled trials involving 182 patients demonstrated non-inferior healing times between AI-enhanced telemedicine and standard outpatient care, with amputation rates decreasing by 8.3% (95% CI: −16.3%, −0.5%) through telemedicine implementation.

7. Quality assurance and standardization

Generative AI applications contribute to quality assurance and standardization efforts in DFU care by providing consistent assessment criteria, standardized documentation formats, and objective performance metrics that enhance care quality across different healthcare settings and providers while addressing significant inter-observer variability that has historically limited wound care consistency.

7.1 Standardized assessment protocols and inter-rater reliability

Vision-language models enable generation of standardized assessment protocols that ensure consistent evaluation criteria across different healthcare providers and settings [20, 21]. Recent validation studies demonstrate achievement of Krippendorff's > 0.8000 for all reliability studies, indicating excellent clinical agreement, while AI systems maintain perfect 100% consistency in repeated assessments compared to significant human inter-rater variability.

Generated assessment protocols include specific measurement techniques, documentation requirements, photographic standards, and evaluation criteria that align with evidence-based guidelines [5]. The CARES4WOUNDS system achieved intra-rater reliability of 0.933–0.994 across 547 images from 28 diabetic foot ulcer patients, establishing robust foundations for standardized wound assessment practices.

The implementation of standardized protocols addresses the critical challenge of subjective variability in wound assessment that has limited treatment consistency across different healthcare providers. AI-enhanced assessment reduces diagnostic variability between clinicians by 60% while improving overall diagnostic accuracy through objective, quantitative measurement approaches.

7.2 Performance monitoring and bias mitigation

Generative models can analyze patterns in treatment outcomes, documentation quality, and adherence to care protocols to identify opportunities for performance improvement while addressing algorithmic bias that may affect care quality for different patient populations. Systematic studies have identified bias in 94 of 152 AI healthcare applications, highlighting the critical importance of continuous monitoring and bias mitigation strategies.

The implementation of comprehensive bias detection frameworks addresses six major bias categories affecting medical AI systems: algorithmic bias from training data or model architecture, selection bias from non-representative populations, measurement bias from inconsistent data collection, temporal bias from changes over time, implicit bias from societal prejudices embedded in data, and confounding bias from unmeasured variables.

Mitigation strategies encompass preprocessing approaches including resampling and data augmentation, in-processing methods using fairness-aware training algorithms, post-processing techniques for output calibration and threshold optimization, and selective deployment strategies that utilize AI where performance is reliable while deferring uncertain cases to human clinicians.

Automated analysis of treatment patterns can identify deviations from evidence-based protocols, highlight successful treatment approaches, and suggest modifications to improve outcomes [9, 10]. This data-driven approach supports clinical decision-making while facilitating adoption of best practices across healthcare teams and reducing disparities in care quality.

8. Regulatory frameworks and clinical implementation

The regulatory landscape for AI-enabled medical devices has undergone dramatic transformation, with comprehensive frameworks emerging to accommodate generative AI innovations while maintaining rigorous safety standards. The FDA's January 2025 Draft Guidance on "Artificial Intelligence-Enabled Device Software Functions" represents the first comprehensive lifecycle management framework for AI medical devices, establishing predetermined change control plans (PCCPs) that allow continuous learning and improvement post-market deployment while maintaining regulatory oversight.

8.1 Current regulatory pathways and approval processes

Over 950 AI/ML-enabled medical devices have received FDA authorization as of 2024, with 76% proceeding through the 510(k) pathway based on substantial equivalence. The Software as Medical Device (SaMD) framework provides clear classification criteria for AI applications in wound care, with most DFU assessment tools qualifying for Class II medical device designation requiring premarket clearance.

The DermaSensor approval in January 2024 established important precedents for AI diagnostic tools in non-specialist settings, demonstrating FDA acceptance of AI systems that can be deployed in primary care rather than requiring specialist oversight. This precedent is particularly relevant for DFU applications, given the need for early detection in primary care settings where specialist expertise may not be readily available.

International regulatory harmonization has accelerated through coordinated efforts between the FDA, European Medicines Agency (EMA), and Health Canada. The EMA AI Workplan 2023–2028 provides a comprehensive strategy across four dimensions: guidance development, AI tool creation, collaboration and training initiatives, and experimental validation protocols. Integration with EU AI Act requirements for high-risk AI systems creates a robust framework emphasizing transparency, accountability, and fundamental rights protection.

8.2 Ethical considerations and synthetic data governance

Ethical considerations for synthetic medical data have received particular attention in recent regulatory guidance, addressing the unique challenges posed by generative AI applications in healthcare. FDA position statements clarify that synthetic data is acceptable for algorithm development but requires extensive real-world validation for regulatory approval, with quality assurance protocols mandating comprehensive documentation and validation procedures.

The regulatory framework specifically addresses bias mitigation as a core requirement, mandating demographic representation reporting, bias testing across subpopulations, performance monitoring by patient groups, and corrective action protocols for identified disparities. This focus is particularly relevant for DFU applications, given that diabetic foot ulcers disproportionately affect underserved populations and require validation across diverse demographic groups.

Quality assurance protocols for synthetic data require documentation of generation methods, fidelity assessment comparing synthetic to real data, utility evaluation for intended medical purposes, and privacy risk assessment. These requirements ensure that generative AI applications maintain clinical relevance while protecting patient privacy and data integrity throughout the development and deployment lifecycle.

9. Future directions and emerging applications

The continued advancement of generative AI presents numerous opportunities for expanding applications in DFU treatment, including integration with emerging technologies, development of more sophisticated modeling approaches, and expansion into new domains of wound care management. Market projections indicate growth from USD 1.8 billion in 2023 to USD 17.2 billion by 2032, with compound annual growth rates of 33–37% reflecting strong industry confidence in the technology's potential.

9.1 Advanced technological integration

Future developments include physics-informed generative models that incorporate biological and physical principles governing wound healing processes [11]. These models could generate more accurate predictions by incorporating mechanistic understanding of tissue repair, inflammatory responses, vascular dynamics, and therapeutic interventions at multiple biological scales.

The integration of hyperspectral imaging capabilities with generative AI promises revolutionary diagnostic potential, enabling bacterial signature identification, tissue viability assessment, and perfusion analysis with unprecedented precision. Advanced diagnostic capabilities under development include fluorescence imaging for real-time bacterial load measurement and 3D wound reconstruction using smartphone cameras for precise volume measurements and healing progression tracking.

Augmented reality applications powered by generative AI could provide real-time guidance for wound care procedures, treatment planning, and patient education. These immersive technologies could enhance clinical training while improving patient understanding of their care requirements through interactive, personalized educational experiences that adapt to individual learning preferences and clinical presentations.

9.2 Long-term vision and societal impact

The long-term vision for generative AI in DFU treatment encompasses comprehensive, personalized care systems that integrate multiple data sources, provide continuous monitoring capabilities, and adapt to individual patient needs while addressing global health disparities. Success in this endeavor requires continued collaboration between technologists, clinicians, regulators, and patients to ensure that AI advancements translate into meaningful improvements in wound healing outcomes and quality of life.

Future breakthrough areas include fully automated wound assessment and monitoring systems, personalized treatment optimization algorithms leveraging genetic and clinical biomarkers, predictive models for amputation risk prevention, and AI-driven drug discovery for wound healing compounds. The integration of wearable sensors and IoT devices with generative AI promises continuous monitoring capabilities with predictive intervention strategies that could prevent complications before they become clinically apparent.

10. Conclusion

The applications of generative AI in diabetic foot ulcer treatment represent a fundamental transformation in wound care delivery, education, and research, with demonstrated clinical validation, regulatory approval pathways, and increasing real-world deployment across diverse healthcare settings. The examined applications provide practical solutions that address longstanding challenges including data scarcity, assessment variability, documentation burden, and treatment personalization while establishing new standards for objective, data-driven wound care.

Diffusion models for synthetic DFU image generation have achieved remarkable clinical fidelity with 70% of generated images being indistinguishable from real wounds by expert clinicians, effectively addressing the chronic shortage of diverse training data while enabling comprehensive educational programs and robust AI system development. Vision-language models provide transformative solutions for automated clinical documentation, achieving 95.34% accuracy in multi-class wound categorization while demonstrating 22% improvement in clinical narrative quality and 50% reduction in documentation time.

Treatment recommendation systems powered by generative AI enable personalized care planning that synthesizes evidence-based protocols with patient-specific factors, achieving 86.9% accuracy in treatment response prediction while demonstrating 18.5% reduction in healing times across diverse patient populations. Predictive modeling applications enable proactive treatment planning through accurate forecasting of healing trajectories and complication risks, with systems achieving 86% accuracy in predicting wound closure within 4 weeks and 91% accuracy in identifying infection risk within 1–2 weeks.

The regulatory landscape has evolved to accommodate AI innovation while maintaining safety standards, with over 950 AI/ML-enabled medical devices receiving FDA authorization and comprehensive international frameworks providing clear pathways for continued development and deployment. The emphasis on bias mitigation, transparency, and continuous monitoring ensures that AI systems serve to reduce rather than exacerbate health disparities while maintaining the highest standards of patient safety and care quality.

The foundation established by current research and clinical validation studies provides a robust platform for the continued evolution of AI-enhanced wound care, with the potential to transform diabetic foot ulcer management from a reactive, experience-based practice to a proactive, data-driven discipline that optimizes outcomes while reducing healthcare costs and improving accessibility to expert-level care across diverse healthcare settings and patient populations.

Acknowledgements

The author thanks the Zivot Limb Preservation Centre, KITE Research Institute at University Health Network, and collaborating institutions for their support in advancing generative AI applications in diabetic foot ulcer treatment. Special recognition is extended to the clinical teams and patients who participated in validation studies that established the clinical utility of these innovative technologies.

Conflict of interest

The author declares no conflict of interest related to the content presented in this chapter. All research was conducted according to ethical guidelines and institutional review board approvals where applicable.

Nomenclature and abbreviations

ADZUS	Attention Diffusion Zero-shot Unsupervised System
AI	artificial intelligence
AUC	area under curve
CNN	convolutional neural network
DDPM	denoising diffusion probabilistic model
DFU	diabetic foot ulcer
DPTD	dependency parse tree depth
EHR	electronic health record
EMA	European Medicines Agency
FDA	Food and Drug Administration
FHIR	Fast Healthcare Interoperability Resources
GAMAN	generative AI-enhanced multi-modal attention network
GAN	generative adversarial network
GPT	generative pre-trained transformer
IoMT	Internet of Medical Things
IoU	Intersection over Union
LLaVA	Large Language and Vision Assistant
LLM	large language model
LoRA	Low-Rank Adaptation
MDR	Medical Device Regulation
PCCP	predetermined change control plan
RGB	red green blue (imaging)
SaMD	Software as Medical Device
SHAP	SHapley Additive exPlanations
UNet	U-Network (architecture)
WIfI	Wound-Ischemia-Foot Infection (classification system)

Author details

Reza Basiri[1,2,3]

1 KITE Research Institute, University Health Network, Toronto, Canada

2 Institute of Biomedical Engineering, University of Toronto, Toronto, Canada

3 Zivot Limb Preservation Centre, Peter Lougheed Centre, Calgary, Canada

*Address all correspondence to: reza.basiri@mail.utoronto.ca

IntechOpen

References

[1] Armstrong DG, Tan T-W, Boulton AJM, Bus SA. Diabetic foot ulcers: A review. JAMA. 2023;**330**(1):62-75

[2] Zhang P, Lu J, Jing Y, Tang S, Zhu D, Bi Y. Global epidemiology of diabetic foot ulceration: A systematic review and meta-analysis. Annals of Medicine. 2020;**49**(2):106-116

[3] Armstrong DG, Swerdlow MA, Armstrong AA, Conte MS, Padula WV, Bus SA. Five year mortality and direct costs of care for people with diabetic foot complications are comparable to cancer. Journal of Foot and Ankle Research. 2020;**13**(1):1-4

[4] Cassidy B, Reeves ND, Pappachan JM, et al. The DFUC 2020 dataset: Analysis towards diabetic foot ulcer detection. touchREVIEWS in Endocrinology. 2021;**17**(1):5-11

[5] Basiri R, Manji K, LeLievre PM, Toole J, Kim F, Khan SS, et al. Protocol for metadata and image collection at diabetic foot ulcer clinics: Enabling research in wound analytics and deep learning. Biomedical Engineering Online. 2024;**23**(1):12

[6] Wang SC, Anderson JAE, Evans R, Woo K, Beland B, Sasseville D, et al. Artificial intelligence in wound care: Diagnostic, assessment and treatment of hard-to-heal wounds. Journal of Wound Care. 2020;**30**(12):962-971

[7] Ohura N, Mitsuno R, Sakisaka M, Terabe Y, Morishige Y, Uchiyama A, et al. Real-time prediction of diabetic foot ulcer healing using artificial intelligence. Wound Repair and Regeneration. 2019;**27**(4):366-371

[8] Smith-Strom H, Igland J, Ostbye T, Tell GS, Hausken MF, Graue M, et al. The effect of telemedicine follow-up care on diabetes-related foot ulcers: A cluster-randomized controlled noninferiority trial. Diabetes Care. 2018;**41**(1):96-103

[9] Cassidy B, Kendrick C, Pappachan JM, O'Shea J, Fernandez CJ, Chacko E, et al. Artificial intelligence for automated detection of diabetic foot ulcers: A real-world proof-of-concept clinical evaluation. Diabetes Research and Clinical Practice. 2023;**205**:110902

[10] Wang L, Pedersen PC, Agu E, Strong DM, Tulu B. Smart diabetic foot ulcer scoring system. Scientific Reports. 2024;**14**(1):12076

[11] Chen RJ, Lu MY, Chen TY, Williamson DFK, Mahmood F. Harnessing the power of synthetic data in healthcare: Innovation, application, and privacy. npj Digital Medicine. 2024;**7**(1):12

[12] Rombach R, Blattmann A, Lorenz D, Esser P, Ommer B. High-resolution image synthesis with latent diffusion models. In: Proceedings of the IEEE/ CVF Conference on Computer Vision and Pattern Recognition. New Orleans, LA, USA: Computer Vision Foundation; 2022. pp. 10684-10695

[13] Packhäuser K, Folle L, Thamm F, Maier A. Generation of anonymous chest radiographs using latent diffusion models for training thoracic abnormality classification systems. Scientific Reports. 2023;**13**(1):11166

[14] Li C, Wong C, Zhang S, Usuyama N, Liu H, Yang J, et al. Llava: Large language and vision assistant. arXiv preprint arXiv:2304.08485. 2023

[15] Zhang X, Zhou C, Wahlberg A, Ahuja N, Xu Y, Sun W, et al. PMC-VQA: Visual instruction tuning for medical visual question answering. arXiv preprint arXiv:2305.10415. 2023

[16] Goyal M, Reeves ND, Rajbhandari S, Spragg J, Yap MH. DFU_QUTNET: Diabetic foot ulcer classification using novel deep convolutional neural network. Multimedia Tools and Applications. 2020;**79**(21-22):15655-15677

[17] Das SK, Roy P, Mirmahboub B, Saha R, Datta A. A feature explainability-based deep learning technique for diabetic foot ulcer identification. Scientific Reports. 2025;**15**(1):780

[18] Basiri R, Manji K, Francois H, Poonja A, Popovic MR, Khan SS. Synthesizing diabetic foot ulcer images with diffusion model. In: Machine Learning and Principles and Practice of Knowledge Discovery in Databases: ECML PKDD 2023. Turin, Italy: Springer; 2023. pp. 448-461

[19] Chan KY, Lau CK, Pang MY, Cheung CH. Artificial intelligence in wound care education: Protocol for a scoping review. JMIR Research Protocols. 2024;**13**(1):e52620

[20] Basiri R, Abedi A, Nguyen C, Popovic MR, Khan SS. Ulcergpt: A multimodal approach leveraging large language and vision models for diabetic foot ulcer image transcription. In: Pattern Recognition: ICPR 2024 International Workshops and Challenges. Kolkata, India: Springer; 2025a. pp. 239-253

[21] Mills JL, Conte MS, Armstrong DG, Pomposelli FB, Schanzer A, Sidawy AN, et al. The society for vascular surgery lower extremity threatened limb classification system: Risk stratification based on wound, ischemia, and foot infection (WIfI). Journal of Vascular Surgery. 2014;**59**(1):220-234

[22] Basiri R, Popovic MR, Khan SS. Multimodal healing phase classification of diabetic foot ulcer using generative adaptive multimodal attention network. 2025 [Preprint]

Chapter 5

Stepping up to the Challenge: Confronting the Global Burden of Diabetic Foot Disease

Hesham Aljohary, Musab Ahmed Murad, Rashad Alfkey and Sherif Elgohary

Abstract

This chapter explores the profound global implications of diabetic foot disease (DFD), a debilitating complication of diabetes that significantly affects individuals, healthcare systems, and societies worldwide. It examines the rising prevalence of DFD and limb loss, particularly in low- and middle-income countries (LMICs), where limited access to prevention and treatment exacerbates the burden. The chapter highlights the substantial healthcare costs associated with diabetic foot management, including wound care, hospital stays, and long-term disability. It also addresses the psychosocial impact, such as reduced workforce productivity, diminished QoL, and increased mortality. By analyzing global disparities and public health challenges, healthcare systems can address inequities in access to diabetic foot care and improve patient outcomes.

Keywords: diabetic foot disease, global diabetes epidemic, amputation rates, morbidity and mortality, socioeconomic impact, healthcare disparities, preventive care, patient education, quality of life

1. Introduction

Diabetes is a chronic metabolic disorder that impacts millions of individuals around the globe and can result in a range of complications affecting multiple bodily systems. Poor circulation and neuropathy are key factors that contribute to the development of DFD, which can lead to infections and, in severe cases, lower-limb loss [1]. The implications of DFD extend beyond physical health; it also presents substantial psychosocial and economic challenges. Patients often face reduced mobility, social isolation, and potential job loss, all of which can lead to economic impact due to extended hospital stays and expensive treatments. In high-income countries (HICs), effective prevention measures and the collaboration of multidisciplinary teams have led to significantly lower rates of DFD and limb loss. People in HICs are more likely to engage in healthy behaviors and have better resources that promote good health [2].

IntechOpen

In contrast, LMICs experience a higher prevalence of DFDs and limb loss, primarily due to inadequate healthcare infrastructure, delayed diagnoses, and a lack of effective preventive measures. Lower income is often linked to reduced healthcare services, leading to worse health outcomes [3]. Structured programs and early diagnosis initiatives play a crucial role in reducing complications and enhancing patient outcomes.

2. Global epidemiology

The incidence of diabetes, along with associated complications, continues to rise. Among these complications, DFDs are linked to increased morbidity and mortality rates [4]. According to the International Diabetes Federation (IDF), approximately 589 million adults aged 20 to 79 are currently living with diabetes, which translates to about 1 in 9 individuals worldwide. Alarmingly, this figure is projected to escalate to 853 million by the year 2050. In 2024 alone, diabetes was responsible for 3.4 million deaths, equating to one death every 6 seconds. The economic impact of diabetes is equally staggering, with healthcare expenditures exceeding USD 1 trillion. As the global prevalence of type 2 diabetes mellitus (T2DM) continues to rise, there is a corresponding increase in the incidence of DFD and related limb loss that has emerged as the leading cause of disability among individuals with diabetes [5]. The highest prevalence of diabetic foot ulcers (DFUs) is observed in North America at 13.0%, followed by Africa (7.2%), Asia (5.5%), Europe (5.1%), and Oceania (3.0%) [6, 7]. The average prevalence across multiple South American countries is about 15% (**Figure 1**) [8].

In 2021, the global prevalence of diabetes was estimated at 10.5%. Notably, this figure was higher in urban areas (12.1%) compared to rural regions (8.3%), and it was also greater in HICs (11.1%) than in LMICs (5.5%) [9]. Approximately 25% of individuals with diabetes (19–34%) will experience DFD at some point during their illness. Studies indicate that the global prevalence of DFUs is around 6.3%, with rates soaring to 13% in North America [10]. The recurrence rates can alarmingly reach as high as 65% within 3 to 5 years [11, 12]. Each year, an estimated 18.6 million individuals with diabetes worldwide will develop a foot ulcer, and about 34%

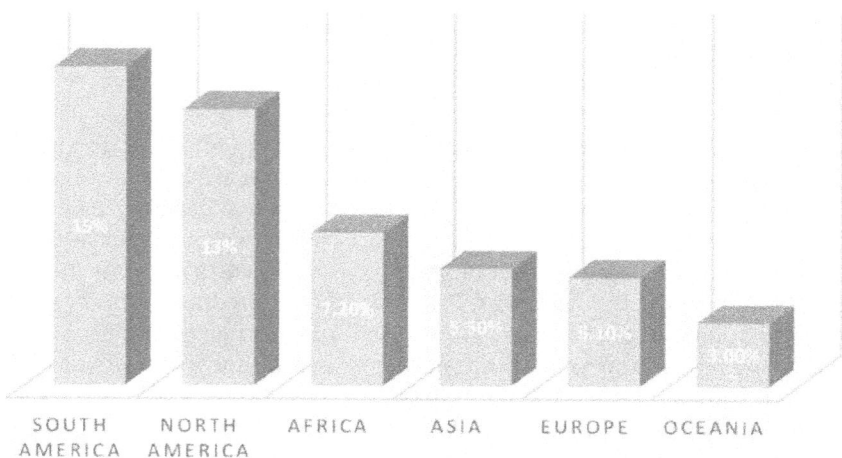

Figure 1.
Regional prevalence of diabetic foot ulcers.

of all people with type 1 or type 2 diabetes will face this complication at some stage in their lives [13, 14]. DFDs are a leading cause of hospital stays among diabetes complications [15].

DFUs contribute significantly to global disability, accounting for roughly 2% of all disability-adjusted life years (DALYs) lost due to diabetes and its complications. Individuals with DFUs experience a marked decline in QoL, with significant reductions in quality-adjusted life years (QALYs). Contributing factors include frequent hospital admissions, persistent pain, limited mobility, and social isolation. The economic impact is considerable, encompassing both direct medical costs and indirect losses such as reduced productivity and long-term disability—often exceeding the financial impact of several major cancers. Moreover, social determinants like income level, race or ethnicity, exacerbate disparities in DFU incidence, outcomes, and availability of team-based foot care, particularly in LMICs [6].

2.1 Mortality

Individuals with DFD can expect a life expectancy that is reduced by 5 years compared to their peers with diabetes. The survival rate following a major amputation is notably lower than the five-year survival rate for patients with many local cancers [14]. The five-year survival rate following the onset of a DFU is approximately 50%, which is significantly lower than the survival rates for many common cancers [16].

Key risk factors associated with mortality in patients with DFD include age, male gender, chronic kidney disease, and the presence of peripheral artery disease (PAD). The combination of both DFD and end-stage renal disease (ESRD) faces a much higher risk of mortality compared to those with ESRD alone. This is due to the combined effects of peripheral artery disease, neuropathy, and systemic inflammation, which are common in both conditions [17]. Furthermore, individuals suffering from DFUs or Charcot foot may experience a reduction in life expectancy of up to 14 years [18]. Recent meta-analyses estimate that approximately 30–40% of patients with DFUs die within 5 years, while the mortality rate exceeds 70% for those who have had major putation. One comprehensive review involving over 120,000 patients reported a 5-year survival rate of just 51% for DFU cases, with cardiovascular disease and infections being the primary causes of death. Moreover, individuals with DFUs experience significantly higher mortality than diabetics without foot ulcers—231 versus 182 deaths per 1000 person-years—underscoring the broader systemic impact of complications such as infection, ischemia, peripheral artery disease, and cardiovascular comorbidities [6, 19–21].

Australian cohort data illustrate a 5-year mortality of 24.6% for people with DFU, increasing to 45.4% at 10 years, with deaths frequently due to chronic kidney disease, cardiovascular disease, sepsis, and multi-organ failure. The mortality rate is lower among neuropathic ulcer patients (16% at 5 years), emphasizing the prognostic impact of ulcer etiology. Additional risk factors for increased mortality include advanced age, peripheral artery disease, chronic kidney disease, prior limb loss, prior cardiovascular events, poor perfusion, ulcer severity, longer ulcer duration, and neuropathy [12, 21].

Prognosis significantly declines following a major lower-limb amputation, with 5-year mortality rates reaching as high as 74%. DFUs often precede limb loss—approximately 20% of moderate to severe DFU cases result in lower extremity amputation, and DFUs are present in about 80% of diabetes-related limb loss (**Figure 2**).

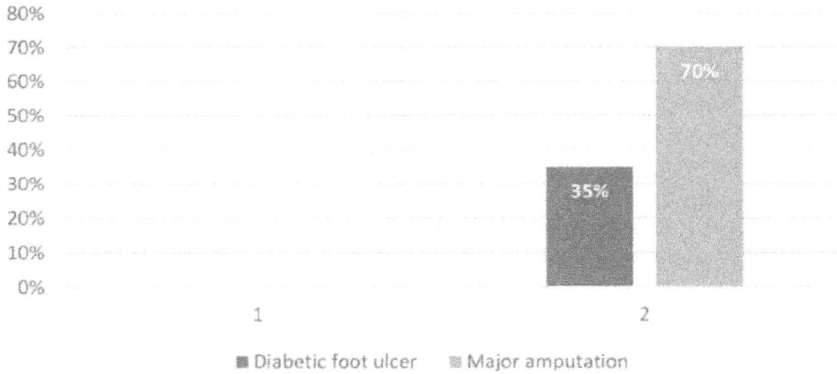

Figure 2.
Five-year mortality rates in diabetic foot ulcer patients vs. major amputation patients (IDF 2024).

2.2 Financial burden

Diabetes mellitus has resulted in health expenditures of at least USD 966 billion worldwide, marking a significant 316% increase over the past 15 years [22]. DFDs impose a significant global burden on both patients and health systems, leading to substantial economic impact across care settings and extended hospital stays. The cost of managing DFD accounts for a major share of healthcare expenditures, surpassing the combined costs of prostate and lung cancers [23].

In the U.S., DFUs represent a major contributor to wound care expenses, with Medicare alone allocating over $6 billion annually for their treatment. DFUs are implicated in approximately 83% of major and 96% of minor lower limb loss, driving substantial treatment costs through repeated hospital stays and extended care. On average, the annual treatment cost per patient is estimated at $8600, with national expenditures reaching into the billions. Although amputation rates among diabetic patients declined by roughly 40% between 2000 and 2009, recent trends show a resurgence, highlighting persistent challenges in prevention and management [20].

In Europe, the average annual cost per patient with DFUs is approximately USD 13,500, highlighting the substantial economic impact of managing the condition. In the United Kingdom, around 0.6% of the National Health Service (NHS) budget is dedicated to DFU care, illustrating the financial variability and complexity associated with addressing DFDs [24].

Hospitalization expenses are the primary contributors to the overall cost of DFU care, particularly for patients undergoing surgical procedures or treatment for infections and complications like osteomyelitis and gangrene. A scoping review covering studies from 2014 to 2024 identified hospitalization as the most substantial cost component in DFU care, with costs escalating in cases requiring surgery—especially limb loss. The review also highlighted wide variations in costs across countries, underscoring the need for standardized care protocols and cost-effective strategies to improve outcomes and reduce financial burden [25].

Out-of-pocket expenses (OOPE) for DFU patients are often financially devastating, particularly in low-income settings where social protection systems are limited. A recent cross-sectional study conducted in South India found that nearly half of the individuals with DFUs incurred catastrophic OOPE, which adversely affected their QoL and complicated disease management [7].

Considering the high costs associated with DFD, interventions aimed at reducing ulcer incidence, accelerating healing, or preventing limb loss offer both clinical and economic benefits. Cost-effectiveness studies suggest that innovative therapies such as platelet-rich plasma (PRP) gel not only enhance health outcomes but also lower treatment expenses, improving quality-adjusted life years (QALYs) and demonstrating potential for substantial healthcare savings [20].

In low-income countries, DFUs place a significant economic impact on healthcare systems and affected individuals. A hospital-based study in northwestern Nigeria estimated the total cost of DFU care at approximately $140,735, with a median cost per patient around $1381.55. Most patients earned less than $100 per month, and out-of-pocket payments covered 90% of expenses, creating severe financial hardship—especially for those who are unemployed or primary earners for their families. The absence of insurance coverage and delayed hospital visits further worsen both clinical outcomes and economic impact [21].

In Iran, DFUs impose a substantial economic impact, with total costs estimated between $8.7 billion and $35 billion—equivalent to 0.59% to 2.41% of the country's GDP. Direct treatment costs account for roughly 20.75% of this figure, while indirect costs, primarily due to productivity losses from premature death and disability, make up nearly 80%. The average hospital stay for DFU patients is 8.1 days, contributing significantly to overall treatment costs. These findings highlight the urgent need for preventive measures and early intervention strategies to reduce both health and economic impacts [26].

In Southeast Asia and tropical regions, DFUs are linked to extended hospital stays and rising treatment costs, which tend to increase with the severity of the condition. A study involving a diverse group of patients in Singapore found that annual treatment costs ranged from approximately $3368 for those receiving ulcer-only care to as much as $30,131 for patients who underwent major limb loss. These high costs are largely driven by prolonged inpatient care and surgical procedures, placing considerable pressure on healthcare systems in these regions [27].

3. Risk factors

Risk factors for DFD include advanced age, being male, having type 2 diabetes, low BMI, hypertension, diabetic retinopathy, and smoking [28]. These can be classified as modifiable or non-modifiable. Modifiable risk factors are those that can be managed through lifestyle changes, medical interventions, or preventive measures, while non-modifiable risk factors, such as gender and age, cannot be altered but must be carefully monitored to reduce their impact.

Non-modifiable risk factors include the duration of diabetes, as longer disease presence heightens the risk of neuropathy and vascular issues. Age is another factor, as older individuals experience reduced healing capacity. Genetics may predispose individuals to poor wound healing and diabetes-related complications, while peripheral neuropathy, which leads to progressive nerve damage, increases the likelihood of unnoticed injuries. Finally, peripheral arterial disease (PAD) restricts blood flow, impairing tissue healing and further complicating DFD management.

Addressing the modifiable risk factors can potentially reduce the risk of DFD, including the need for limb amputations, ultimately enhancing their quality of life [29]. Glycemic control and smoking are the only modifiable risk factors consistently associated with DFD. Poor glycemic control accelerates nerve and vascular damage, increasing the likelihood of foot ulcers and complications, while smoking impairs circulation, delaying wound healing and raising the risk of severe infections. Other modifiable risk factors include a sedentary lifestyle, which increases obesity risk and poor circulation. Wearing improper footwear can cause pressure sores and injuries, while uncontrolled hypertension and hyperlipidemia can worsen vascular complications. Additionally, delayed wound care, often resulting from poor hygiene or neglect, can lead to ulcer formation [29]. Cultural beliefs and practices greatly influence how individuals approach the management of diabetes and foot care. Some communities may rely on traditional healing methods, which can sometimes hinder timely medical intervention. Moreover, there is a stigma surrounding diabetes-related amputations that may deter patients from seeking necessary care.

Geographic factors also play a significant role in the management of DFDs. Environmental conditions further exacerbate the severity of complications associated with DFDs. For instance, tropical climates can lead to intensified wound infections due to high temperatures and humidity, while colder regions can worsen peripheral circulation [3].

4. Burden on healthcare systems in low- and middle-income countries (LMICs)

The lack of sufficient healthcare infrastructure in LMICs results in delayed diagnoses and ineffective treatment. Financial barriers also deter patients from seeking preventive care, as necessary medical supplies—such as protective footwear and wound dressings—are either too expensive or unavailable. Additionally, cultural perspectives and reliance on traditional medicine may contribute to postponing medical intervention, heightening the risk of severe infections. DFDs impose a substantial economic burden on healthcare systems, driving up costs associated with hospitalizations, advanced treatments, and long-term care [30]. Furthermore, the economic impact of treatment costs and job loss can intensify stress, leading to strained family dynamics and relationships. Caregivers also experience emotional and physical strain as they play a vital role in managing the patient's condition [31]. The decrease in productivity resulting from unemployment or sick leave due to foot disease management represents an additional financial burden on families, relatives, friends, and communities in low-income countries. This cost is often overlooked and not fully quantified [32].

DFDs pose a serious challenge to healthcare systems in LMICs due to high prevalence and resource constraints. The absence of dedicated diabetic foot clinics in many hospitals results in delayed diagnoses, inadequate wound management, and increased amputation rates. A shortage of trained professionals, including podiatrists and wound care specialists, exacerbates the issue, while the lack of advanced diagnostic tools, specialized footwear, and essential medications further worsens patient outcomes. Overcrowded healthcare facilities and prolonged hospital stays for DFD patients place additional pressure on already underfunded health systems, diverting resources from other critical services. Moreover, the financial burden of treating DFDs—encompassing hospital stays, surgeries, antibiotic therapy, and long-term wound care—can lead to overwhelming healthcare expenses, particularly for families in low-income communities. The high costs associated with limb loss, such as surgical procedures, rehabilitation, and prosthetic needs, further exacerbate the economic impact. Indirect expenses, such as loss of income due to disability and the necessity for caregivers to leave their jobs, only add to the economic challenges faced by affected individuals and their families. Other barriers include long travel distances, delays in referrals and treatment, fragmented care systems, uninformed amputation recommendations, and insufficient training programs. Additionally, many foot care services are provided by nurses rather than dedicated specialists, highlighting the urgent need for systemic healthcare improvements and expanded professional training opportunities (**Table 1**) [33].

4.1 Amputation in diabetic foot diseases

DFUs are a critical precursor to diabetes-related amputations, with studies indicating that they precede approximately 85% of such cases [34]. It's estimated that 40–70% of non-traumatic lower-limb amputations are linked to DFD [35]. The mortality rate for people who undergo major lower limb amputation in DFD is more than 50% in 5 years [36]. DFD-like foot ulcers, infections, and peripheral artery disease (PAD) continue to drive high hospital admission rates. These conditions often precede amputations and highlight gaps in early intervention and preventive care [5]. Unlike major amputations, minor amputations (e.g., toe or partial foot) have shown stable or even increasing trends in some regions. This could reflect improved efforts to prevent major amputations, but also indicates ongoing challenges in managing advanced DFD [5, 37].

Amputations contribute to long-term healthcare expenses, including prosthetics, follow-up care, and treatment of complications. In 2020, the total direct medical costs of major amputations in the U.S. were estimated at $13.4 billion, with additional indirect costs from lost productivity [38]. In LMICs, amputation rates are disproportionately higher, with up to 20% of DFU cases resulting in lower-limb amputations. The burden of DFDs is further intensified in regions with rising diabetes incidence, such as South Asia, Sub-Saharan Africa, and parts of the Middle East and North Africa (MENA). Studies highlight prevalence rates exceeding 10% in some LMICs. Individuals with lower socioeconomic status often experience higher rates of chronic diseases such as diabetes, cardiovascular diseases, and certain cancers. This is due to a combination of factors, including poorer living conditions and higher levels of stress [2]. Adults living in LMICs have higher rates of diabetes (**Table 1**) [39].

4.2 Psychosocial and economic impacts

DFDs have profound medical, psychological, and financial effects on individuals, their families, and society. They contribute to a high risk of infections, lower-limb

Aspect	LMICs	HICs
DM Prevalence	Rapidly increasing	Stabilizing
Registry Data	Sparse and inconsistent	Robust registries
DFD	Higher rates/ late diagnosis	Lower rates
Amputation Rates	Up to 25 times higher	Significantly lower
Access to Care	Limited access	Broad access
Footwear	Often unavailable	Widely available

Table 1.
Comparison between low- and middle-income countries (LMICs) and high-income countries (HICs).

loss, disability, diminished QoL, increased mortality rates, and a significant economic impact on healthcare systems [30]. The psychosocial impacts of DFD are profound, stemming from restricted mobility, chronic pain, and the social stigma associated with visible wounds or limb loss. Many patients struggle with depression, anxiety, and a diminished QoL as they navigate prolonged treatments, frequent hospital visits, and the constant risk of amputation. These challenges often lead to social isolation, reduced work productivity, and increased dependence on caregivers, further intensifying their mental health burdens [40].

5. Prevention strategies for diabetic foot disease

Reducing the global prevalence of DFD is essential for minimizing complications and improving patient outcomes. It necessitates a comprehensive, multi-level approach focused on early diagnosis and effective management. Moreover, increasing public awareness through educational campaigns on proper foot care and glycemic control can empower patients to take proactive steps in reducing their risk of developing DFDs. The training of healthcare professionals, particularly in LMICs, can enhance patient outcomes. Additionally, the development of cost-effective treatments, such as locally produced therapeutic footwear and affordable wound care solutions, can improve accessibility for marginalized populations [41]. These strategies incorporate medical, lifestyle, and educational approaches: [42].

- Medical measures include regular foot screenings—annually for all diabetics and more frequently for high-risk patients. Risk assessment tests, such as monofilament (10 g), vibration perception, and ankle-brachial index (ABI), help identify potential issues early. Maintaining optimal glycemic control, with a focus on HbA1c levels, plays a critical role in prevention.

- Lifestyle interventions emphasize daily foot inspections, proper footwear (e.g., custom orthotics), and good hygiene, including regular washing and moisturizing. Patients should avoid foot trauma from hot water bottles, heating pads, and walking barefoot. Additionally, smoking cessation and reducing alcohol consumption are vital, as smoking doubles the risk of amputation.

- Education & community programs are pivotal in preventing DFD. Patient education raises awareness about foot care, early complication detection, and the importance of glycemic control. Structured programs have proven to reduce DFU risk by 30–60%, reinforcing the need for proactive prevention efforts. Additionally, awareness campaigns, such as World Diabetes Day, promote prevention and early intervention efforts worldwide.

5.1 Successful national and international initiatives in diabetic foot care

A range of international and national initiatives have made substantial contributions toward alleviating the burden of DFD through structured training, early detection, and improved healthcare policies.

5.1.1 International initiatives

The global collaboration through partnerships between international organizations, healthcare institutions, and policymakers is essential in driving impactful change. Initiatives like the WHO Global Diabetes Compact and the International Working Group on the Diabetic Foot (IWGDF) promote standardized guidelines and best practices that can be implemented across various healthcare settings [43].

- The International Working Group on the Diabetic Foot (IWGDF) develops policies for diabetic foot care. They publish evidence-based guidelines every 4 years that cover prevention strategies, infection management, offloading techniques, and screening for peripheral artery disease (PAD).

- International Diabetes Federation (IDF) – Leads advocacy, education, and research, influencing healthcare policies worldwide. The IDF Diabetes Atlas provides global data on diabetes prevalence, healthcare costs, and mortality rates.

- WHO Global Diabetes Compact – Promotes structured diabetic foot care in national healthcare policies to enhance access to prevention and treatment.

- Diabetes Foot Network (Africa & Middle East) – Strengthens regional collaborations to advance podiatry training, early detection, and cost-effective wound care solutions.

5.1.2 National programs

Many low- and middle-income countries have faced unique obstacles in diabetic foot care, leading to innovative approaches in training, accessibility, and policy integration [44]. Community-based initiatives, such as mobile clinics and outreach programs, play a crucial role in providing healthcare services in rural areas.

- Step-by-Step Program (Tanzania & India) – Structured training for healthcare professionals has resulted in a 50% reduction in amputation rates in participating regions [45].

- Save the Diabetic Foot Project (Brazil) – Integrating diabetic foot clinics with early screening efforts has led to a 78% decrease in lower-limb amputations over 9 years.

- Diabetic Footcare Pathway (United Kingdom) – A multidisciplinary approach emphasizing early intervention has significantly lowered hospital admissions for DFUs [33].

6. Future directions

Technological innovations, including AI-based diagnostics, wearable glucose monitors, and telemedicine services, are transforming the early detection of foot complications. Recent advancements in early detection technologies, including smart socks, AI algorithms, and wound healing biomarkers, are enhancing new treatments such as stem cell therapy, growth factors, bioengineered skin substitutes, and negative pressure wound therapy (NPWT).

AI models analyze foot images to detect early signs of ulcers, infections, or tissue damage. AI-enhanced thermal cameras detect temperature differences that may indicate inflammation or pre-ulcerative conditions [46]. Machine learning algorithms assess patient data (e.g., glucose levels, neuropathy, foot pressure) to predict the likelihood of DFU development. AI can generate individualized risk profiles to guide preventive care and monitoring [47]. It can be used to classify wound severity and segment wound areas from clinical images. Smartphone Applications allow patients to monitor foot health at home, reducing the need for frequent clinic visits, and may suggest treatment plans based on wound type, size, and healing progress [48].

Innovations in vascular and surgical procedures—like endovascular revascularization, 3D-printed orthotics, and Charcot foot reconstruction—along with antimicrobial methods such as antibiotic-coated implants and phage therapy, are greatly improving patient outcomes. Future developments in podiatry include using telemedicine for remote monitoring of foot ulcers, implementing AI-driven diagnostic tools, and providing affordable treatment options.

7. Conclusions

As life expectancy for individuals with diabetes continues to rise, the prevalence of DFD is also increasing, leading to a higher rate of lower extremity amputations. To mitigate this trend, effective preventive strategies are essential, including strict glycemic control, regular foot screenings, patient education, and early intervention for foot complications. Expanding access to podiatric care, multidisciplinary management approaches, and advanced wound care techniques can further help reduce the incidence of DFD and lower extremity amputations. Strengthening public health initiatives and healthcare policies focused on diabetic foot prevention is crucial to improving long-term outcomes for diabetic patients.

Author details

Hesham Aljohary[1*], Musab Ahmed Murad[1], Rashad Alfkey[2] and Sherif Elgohary[3]

1 Acute care Surgery Department, Hamad Medical Corporation, Doha, Qatar

2 Surgery Department HMC, Director of Wound Services, Doha, Qatar

3 Qatar University, Doha, Qatar

*Address all correspondence to: heljohary@hamad.qa

IntechOpen

References

[1] van Netten JJ, Bus SA, Apelqvist J, et al. Definitions and criteria for diabetic foot disease. Diabetes & Metabolic Research and Reviews. 2019;**36**(S1):e3268. DOI: 10.1002/dmrr.3268

[2] Dagenais GR, Gerstein HC, Zhang X, McQueen M, Lear S, Lopez-Jaramillo P, et al. Variations in diabetes prevalence in low-, middle-, and high-income countries: Results from the prospective urban and rural epidemiological study. Diabetes Care. 2016;**39**(5):780-787. DOI: 10.2337/dc15-2338

[3] Thaniyath TA. Diabetic foot syndrome: Risk factors, clinical assessment, and advances in diagnosis. In: Zubair M, Ahmad J, Malik A, Talluri MR, editors. Diabetic Foot Ulcer. Singapore: Springer; 2021. DOI: 10.1007/978-981-15-7639-3_11

[4] Daniyal, Nawaz A, Zaidi A, Elsayed B, Jemmieh K, Eledrisi M. Perspective chapter: Epidemiology and risk factors of diabetic foot ulcer. In: Diabetic Foot Ulcers - Pathogenesis, Innovative Treatments and AI Applications. London, UK: IntechOpen; 2024. DOI: 10.5772/intechopen.1004009

[5] Lazzarini PA, Cramb SM, Golledge J, Morton JI, Magliano DJ, Van Netten JJ. Global trends in the incidence of hospital admissions for diabetes-related foot disease and amputations: A review of national rates in the 21st century. Diabetologia. Feb 2023;**66**(2):267-287. DOI: 10.1007/s00125-022-05845-9. Epub 2022 Dec 13

[6] Haile KE, Asgedom YS, Azeze GA, Amsalu AA, Gebrekidan AY, Kassie GA. Diabetic foot: A systematic review and meta-analysis on its prevalence and associated factors among patients with diabetes mellitus in a sub-Saharan Africa. Diabetes Research and Clinical Practice. 2025;**220**:111975. DOI: 10.1016/j.diabres.2024.111975. Epub 2025 Jan 4

[7] Bodhare T, Bele S, Balakumaran B, Ramji M, Gavin Francis J, Shalini V, et al. Health costs and quality of life among diabetic foot ulcer patients in South India: A cross-sectional study. Cureus. 2025;**17**(3):e79950. DOI: 10.7759/cureus.79950

[8] López-de-Andrés A et al. Diabetic foot in Latin America: Prevalence and outcomes in hospitalized patients with diabetes mellitus. Journal of Clinical Medicine. 2018;7(8):219. DOI: 10.3390/jcm7080219

[9] Sun H, Saeedi P, Karuranga S, Pinkepank M, Ogurtsova K, Duncan BB, et al. IDF diabetes atlas: Global, regional, and country-level diabetes prevalence estimates for 2021 and projections for 2045. Diabetes Research and Clinical Practice. 2022;**183**:109119

[10] Cortes-Penfield NW, Armstrong DG, Brennan MB, Fayfman M, Ryder JH, Tan T-W, et al. Evaluation and management of diabetes-related foot infections. Clinical Infectious Diseases. 2023;**77**(3):e1-e13. DOI: 10.1093/cid/ciad255

[11] McDermott K, Fang M, Boulton AJM, Selvin E, Hicks CW. Etiology, epidemiology, and disparities in the burden of diabetic foot ulcers. Diabetes Care. 2023;**46**(1):209-221. DOI: 10.2337/dci22-0043

[12] OuYang H, Yang J, Wan H, Huang J, Yin Y. Effects of different treatment measures on the efficacy of diabetic foot ulcers: A network meta-analysis.

Frontiers in Endocrinology (Lausanne).
2024;**15**:1452192. DOI: 10.3389/
fendo.2024.1452192

[13] Zhang Y, Lazzarini PA, McPhail SM,
van Netten JJ, Armstrong DG,
Pacella RE. Global disability burdens
of diabetes-related lower-extremity
complications in 1990 and 2016. Diabetes
Care. 2020;**43**(5):964-974. DOI: 10.2337/
dc19-1614

[14] Armstrong DG, Boulton AJM,
Bus SA. Diabetic foot ulcers and their
recurrence. The New England Journal of
Medicine. 2017;**376**(24):2367-2375

[15] Rusu A, Roman G, Stancu B, Bala C.
The burden of diabetic foot ulcers
on hospital admissions and costs in
Romania. Journal of Clinical Medicine.
2025;**14**(4):1248. DOI: 10.3390/
jcm14041248

[16] Armstrong DG, Swerdlow MA,
Armstrong AA. Five-year mortality
and direct costs of care for people
with diabetic foot complications
are comparable to cancer. Journal of
Foot and Ankle Research. 2020;**13**:16.
DOI: 10.1186/s13047-020-00383-2

[17] Ndip A, Lavery LA, Boulton AJM.
Diabetic foot disease in people with
advanced nephropathy and those
on renal dialysis. Current Diabetes
Reports. 2010;**10**:283-290. DOI: 10.1007/
s11892-010-0128-0

[18] van Baal J, Hubbard R, Game F,
Jeffcoate W. Mortality associated with
acute Charcot foot and neuropathic
foot ulceration. Diabetes Care.
2010;**33**(5):1086-1089. DOI: 10.2337/
dc09-1428

[19] Chen L, Sun S, Gao Y, Ran X.
Global mortality of diabetic foot ulcer:
A systematic review and meta-analysis
of observational studies. Diabetes,

Obesity & Metabolism. 2023;**25**(1):36-45.
DOI: 10.1111/dom.14840. Epub 2022 Sep 4

[20] Dhatariya K, Abbas ZG. 7 regions
foot ulcer costs study group. Estimated
costs of treating two standardised
diabetes-related foot ulcers of different
severity - a comparison of 7 global
regions. Diabetes Research and Clinical
Practice. 2025;**221**:112036. DOI: 10.1016/j.
diabres.2025.112036. Epub 2025 Feb 14

[21] Muhammad FY, Pedro LM,
Suleiman HH, Uloko AE, Gezawa ID,
Adenike E, et al. Cost of illness of
diabetic foot ulcer in a resource limited
setting: A study from northwestern
Nigeria. Journal of Diabetes and
Metabolic Disorders. 2018;**17**(2):93-99.
DOI: 10.1007/s40200-018-0344-8

[22] Miller EM. Using continuous
glucose monitoring in clinical practice.
Clinical Diabetes. 2020;**38**(5):429-438.
DOI: 10.2337/cd20-0043

[23] Kerr M, Barron E, Chadwick P,
Evans T, Kong WM, Rayman G, et al. The
cost of diabetic foot ulcers and amputations
to the National Health Service in England.
Diabetic Medicine. 2019;**36**(8):995-1002.
DOI: 10.1111/dme.13973

[24] Waibel FWA, Uçkay I, Soldevila-
Boixader L, Sydler C, Gariani K.
Current knowledge of morbidities and
direct costs related to diabetic foot
disorders: A literature review. Frontiers
in Endocrinology. 2024;**14**:1323315.
DOI: 10.3389/fendo.2023.1323315

[25] Russo S, Landi S, Simoni S. Cost-
effectiveness analysis for managing
diabetic foot ulcer (DFU) in USA:
Platelet-rich plasma (PRP) vs standard
of care (SoC). ClinicoEconomics and
Outcomes Research. 2025;**17**:157-169.
DOI: 10.2147/CEOR.S496616

[26] Hashempour R, MirHashemi S,
Mollajafari F, Damiri S, ArabAhmadi A,

Raei B. Economic burden of diabetic foot ulcer: A case of Iran. BMC Health Services Research. 2024;**24**(1):363. DOI: 10.1186/s12913-024-10873-9

[27] Lo ZJ, Surendra NK, Saxena A, Car J. Clinical and economic burden of diabetic foot ulcers: A 5-year longitudinal multi-ethnic cohort study from the tropics. International Wound Journal. 2021;**18**(3):375-386. DOI: 10.1111/iwj.13540. Epub 2021 Jan 26

[28] Leone S, Pascale R, Vitale M, Esposito S. Epidemiology of diabetic foot. Infezioni in Medicina. 2012;**20**(Suppl. 1):8-13

[29] Rossboth S, Lechleitner M, Oberaigner W. Risk factors for diabetic foot complications in type 2 diabetes—A systematic review. Endocrinology, Diabetes & Metabolism. 2020;**4**(1):e00175. DOI: 10.1002/edm2.175

[30] Apelqvist J. Diagnostics and treatment of the diabetic foot. Endocrine. 2012;**41**(3):384-397. DOI: 10.1007/s12020-012-9619-x

[31] Costa D, Ielapi N, Caprino F, Giannotta N, Sisinni A, Abramo A, et al. Social aspects of diabetic foot: A scoping review. Social Sciences. 2022;**11**:149. DOI: 10.3390/socsci11040149

[32] Cavanagh P, Attinger C, Abbas ZG, Bal A, Rojas N, Xu ZR. Cost of treating diabetic foot ulcers in five different countries. Diabetes & Metabolic Research and Reviews. 2012;**28**:107-111

[33] Abbas ZG, Archibald LK. Challenges for management of the diabetic foot in Africa: Doing more with less. International Wound Journal. 2007;**4**(4):305-313. DOI: 10.1111/j.1742-481X.2007.00376.x

[34] Chamberlain RC, Fleetwood K, Wild SH, Colhoun HM, Lindsay RS, Petrie JR, et al. Foot ulcer and risk of lower limb amputation or death in people with diabetes: A national population-based retrospective cohort study. Diabetes Care. 2022;**45**(1):83-91. DOI: 10.2337/dc21-1596

[35] Meffen A, Rutherford MJ, Sayers RD, Houghton JSM, Bradbury N, Gray LJ. Regional variation in non-traumatic major lower limb amputation in England: Observational study of linked primary and secondary care data. BJS Open. 2025;**9**(2):zraf004. DOI: 10.1093/bjsopen/zraf004

[36] Huang Y-Y, Lin C-W, Yang H-M, Hung S-Y, Chen I-W. Survival and associated risk factors in patients with diabetes and amputations caused by infectious foot gangrene. Journal of Foot and Ankle Research. 2018;**11**:1

[37] Valabhji J, Barron E, Vamos EP, Dhatariya K, Game F, Kar P, et al. Temporal trends in lower-limb major and minor amputation and revascularization procedures in people with diabetes in England during the COVID-19 pandemic. Diabetes Care. 2021;**44**(6):e133-e135. DOI: 10.2337/dc20-2852

[38] Lago S, Cantarero D, Rivera B, et al. Socioeconomic status, health inequalities, and non-communicable diseases: A systematic review. Journal of Public Health. 2018;**26**(1):1-14. DOI: 10.1007/s10389-017-0850-z

[39] Liang S, An W, Sun M, et al. Association between socioeconomic status and the triglyceride glucose index: A cross-sectional study based on NHANES 2007-2016. BMC Public Health. 2025;**25**:934. DOI: 10.1186/s12889-025-22085-9

[40] Beverly EA, Smaldone A. Psychosocial and educational implications of diabetic foot complications. In: Veves A, Giurini JM, Schermerhorn ML, editors. The Diabetic Foot. Contemporary Diabetes. Cham: Humana; 2024. DOI: 10.1007/978-3-031-55715-6_30

[41] Mehndiratta A, Mishra SC, Bhandarkar P, Chhatbar K, Cluzeau F, Doctors PC, et al. Increasing identification of foot at risk of complications in patients with diabetes: A quality improvement project in an urban primary health Centre in India. BMJ Open Quality. 2020;**9**(3):e000893. DOI: 10.1136/bmjoq-2019-000893

[42] Kaminski MR, Golledge J, Lasschuit JWJ, Schott KH, Charles J, Cheney J, et al. Australian guideline on prevention of foot ulceration: Part of the 2021 Australian evidence-based guidelines for diabetes-related foot disease. Journal of Foot and Ankle Research. 2022;**15**(1):53. DOI: 10.1186/s13047-022-00534-7

[43] World Health Organization. The Global Diabetes Compact - Progress in Supporting its Workstreams: Technical Report. Geneva, Switzerland: WHO; 2024. Licence: CC BY-NC-SA 3.0 IGO

[44] Pendsey S, Abbas ZG. The step-by-step program for reducing diabetic foot problems: A model for the developing world. Current Diabetes Reports. 2007;**7**(6):425-428. DOI: 10.1007/s11892-007-0071-x

[45] Gregg EW, Buckley J, Ali MK, Davies J, Flood D, Mehta R, et al. Improving health outcomes of people with diabetes: Target setting for the WHO global diabetes compact. The Lancet. 2023;**401**(10384):1302-1312. DOI: 10.1016/S0140-6736(23)00001-6

[46] Gurjarpadhye AA, Parekh MB, Dubnika A, Rajadas J, Inayathullah M. Infrared imaging tools for diagnostic applications in dermatology. SM Journal Clinical and Medical Imaging. 2015;**1**(1):1-5. Epub 2015 Nov 20

[47] Oei CW, Chan YM, Zhang X, Leo KH, Yong E, Chong RC, et al. Risk prediction of diabetic foot amputation using machine learning and explainable artificial intelligence. Journal of Diabetes Science and Technology. 2025;**19**(4):1008-1022. DOI: 10.1177/19322968241228606. Epub 2024 Jan 30

[48] Debong F, Mayer H, Kober J. Real-world assessments of mySugr Mobile health app. Diabetes Technology & Therapeutics. 2019;**21**(S2):S235-S240. DOI: 10.1089/dia.2019.0019

Edited by Alok Raghav

The Edited Volume, *Diabetic Foot - Advanced Methods of Management,* is a collection of peer-reviewed research chapters that offers a comprehensive overview of recent developments in endocrinology. The book comprises single chapters authored by various researchers and edited by experts active in this research area. All chapters are complete but united under a common research study topic. This publication aims to provide a comprehensive overview of the latest research efforts by international authors in endocrinology, opening new avenues for further development.

Published in London, UK
© 2025 IntechOpen
© vsijan / nightcafe.studio

IntechOpen

ISBN 978-1-83635-371-3

9 781836 353713

www.ingramcontent.com/pod-product-compliance
Lightning Source LLC
Chambersburg PA
CBHW081336190326
41458CB00018B/6015